A CHAPLAIN
THE BUSII

SURVIVING
HO$PICE

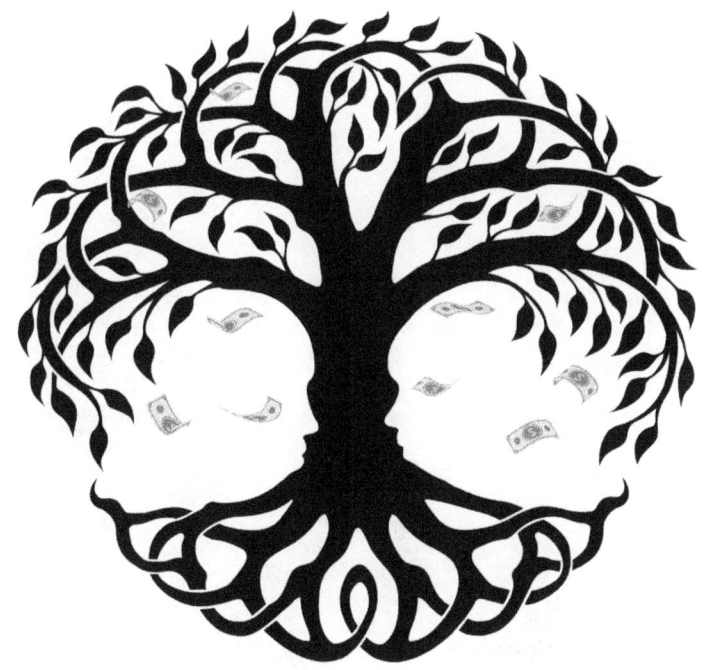

AND HOW TO FIND A
TRUSTWORTHY PROVIDER

MARYCLAIRE TORINUS

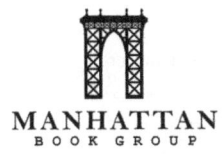

Surviving Hospice: A Chaplain's Journey Into The Business Of Dying.
Copyright © 2023 by Maryclaire Torinus. All rights reserved.

No part of this book may be used or reproduced in any manner whatsoever without written permission, except in the case of brief quotations embodied in critical articles and reviews. For more information, e-mail all inquiries to info@manhattanbookgroup.com.

Manhattan Book Group Publishers
447 Broadway 2nd Floor, #354
New York, NY 10013, USA
1.800.767.0531 www.manhattanbookgroup.com

Printed in the United States of America
ISBN-13: 978-1-960142-55-9

Dedicated to the Eternal Word,

To the Word made flesh,

And to the Creative Spirit who inspired my words and sustained my passion for the years of writing that would lie ahead of me.

"When my fingers knew better than I as they hovered over the keyboard for a better word, what was that—but divine inspiration."
Author unknown

In memory of Mark,
My most fervent ally,
My eternal soulmate.
His spiritual guidance during the writing of this
narrative and whisperings of support could be
sensed from the other side of the Thin Veil.

To my amazing children,
Who challenged me and encouraged this project. They read
early chapters and provided astute insight even as their own
lives were absorbed with family, careers, and service.
Nathan, Sarah, and Annie,
I love you so much.

To Cynthia and Caitlin,
My loving daughters-in-law who have enriched
our family with their loving presence.

To James, Juliette, and Luke, my beloved grandchildren,
When I feel adrift some days without Mark, thoughts of you
ground me. Your kindness and fun-filled personalities restore
my soul with joy, laughter, never-ending wonder, and hope.

For my dedicated and caring former hospice colleagues.
To the families of my deceased patients, it was my privilege to partner
your loved ones through the transition of dying and rebirth.
To those professionals in the hospice industry who
place patients as their primary stakeholders.
To future consumers of the hospice benefit, we will
strive to take the money out of medicine.

Contents

Foreword ix
Preface xiii
Introduction xix

PART ONE
Spiritual Stories of Crossing the Threshold

Going Back 3
The First Year 9
Love and Delight 15
On-Call 23
John 29
A Bullshit Barometer 39
Spirituality and Religion 43
Hell is in Your Mind 49
Schizophrenia 53
Dark Nights 59
Passing Through the Thin Veil 65
Secrets Lie in Shadows 69
A Day Away from Death 75
The Card 85
Martha 91
Defiance 95
What's in a Name? 103

Koda 107
Water, Wind, and Gulls 115
Nature of the Divine 121
Helen 127
Visions and Signs 135
A Company Ruse Backfired 145
The Quantum Leap 153
Morphine, Myths, and George..161
A Gold Mine...167
Let Them Eat Cake...175
There's No Place Like Home 181
Lessons and Insights..185
Afterword..189

PART TWO
How To Make What's Invisible, Visible

How to Find a Trustworthy Provider..195
Qualities of a Reputable Provider 203
Behind the Window Dressing 209

PART THREE
Helping Hospice Return To Its Roots

Dying for Dollars..217
Weak Oversight Breeds Neglect 223
The US Government Sounds an Alarm...................................... 229
Next Steps.. 235
Epilogue: The Moral of the Story 241

Questions for the Chaplain 243
Acknowledgements..251
Notes 255
Index 263

Foreword

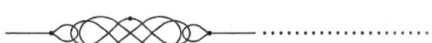

I FIRST MET MARYCLAIRE TORINUS AFTER COMING ACROSS HER WEBsite and learning about her work as a hospice chaplain. She was writing a book about the harm caused by the changing business structure of the hospice industry. My experience with for-profit hospices was as a volunteer, and as the founder and president of the Hospice Volunteer Association (HVA), I had also witnessed a decline in the quality of care from several different perspectives. And what was most troubling was that so much of it seemed directly related to the rising number of for-profit hospices (while nonprofit hospices were decreasing.)

Over time, I have seen my role as a volunteer becoming more limited due to increased regulation driven by the recommendations of corporate lawyers. In early 2008, our association saw an urgent need for the Health Insurance Portability and Accountability Act (HIPAA) for volunteer programs. So, I developed the Patient Data Vault (PDV) software that hospices use to manage their volunteer programs and facilitate reporting that is HIPAA-compliant and meets Medicare requirements.

The most concerning aspect of that restrictive regulation was the premise by corporate lawyers that hospice volunteers should not be permitted to document what occurred during their patient visits. Consequently, the volunteer was only allowed to check generic boxes as to the type of service that was provided, but they could not describe what the patient may have conveyed to them during the appointment for fear of a lawsuit.

As the software began to get greater use in the hospice community, I observed that some hospices were restricting volunteers access to patient data. Zealous administrators and lawyers have created a double standard between volunteers and clinical staff when it comes to providing information that would allow volunteers to best serve the patients. The claim was that it was necessary for HIPAA compliance; however, HIPAA law specifically states that compliance should not sacrifice the quality of care for patients.

Such restrictions imposed on patient data is contrary to the congressional mandate that hospice volunteers are an integral part of the hospice's Interdisciplinary Team (IDT). When Congress established the Medicare Hospice Benefit in 1982, it stipulated that the Conditions of Participation (CoPs) mandated that volunteers must provide administrative or direct patient care in an amount that, at a minimum, equals 5 percent of the total patient care hours expended by all paid hospice employees and contract staff.

Unfortunately, the use of volunteers declined 45 percent, as reflected by the 5 percent metric, from 9.4 percent in 2003 to 5.2 percent in 2014. Coincidentally, the number of for-profit hospices increased by 44 percent over that same period. This is a logical correlation given that for-profit hospices are more likely to target the minimum 5 percent requirement even though a higher target would increase their overall staffing and raise the quality of care at virtually no additional cost.

It's important to note that volunteers were the driving force behind the grassroots establishment of the concept of hospice when it first started. As well, the growing awareness of how hospitals were treating the dying in the mid-70s inspired idealistic nurses, clergy, and volunteers to come forward and help launch hospice as a necessary health care reform. In the 1980s, the concept of hospice care began to resonate with the public and inspired lay people and healthcare professionals alike to place themselves at the disposal of nonprofit hospice providers even though they had just finished eight-hour shifts at their own jobs.

Fast forward thirty years to witness the dramatic changes we observe in the hospice industry today. The end-of-life care environment has transitioned from hospice organizations which began as nonprofit providers and driven by the altruism of lay volunteers to a substantial financial enterprise that is driven by big profit margins.

The unfortunate result of this transition has directly impacted patients and families. I'm not surprised by what Maryclaire observed in her own for-profit company and I agree with what she has shared in this illuminating book: there are less resources available to serve patient needs, less hospice staff to cover the census and provide for the quality and time patients deserve, a reduction in personal fulfillment by employees, and many seasoned and caring professionals are leaving for-profit hospices because the type of care they once provided is no longer possible.

The resources provided in part two of *Surviving Hospice: A Chaplain's Journey into the Business of Dying* will help consumers make informed decisions for the critical choice that patients and their families have for selecting a hospice and ensuring a shot at having a good dying experience. There are no "do-overs" in this business.

Maryclaire Torinus beautifully weaves her own life story with her experiences as a hospice insider who cared for her dying patients until the last moments of their lives. The economic discoveries she makes on her spiritual journey that affected the well-being of her patients and the staff will help you to understand the important nuances associated with assessing and selecting the best hospice for you, whether it be nonprofit or for-profit.

The extremely useful interview tools will guide you step-by-step on how to search for crucial hospice information like a pro; and in the process, clear up why "all hospices are not the same."

Greg Schneider
Founder & President, Hospice Volunteer Association
Founding Director & CEO/CTO, Hospice Educators Affirming Life (HEAL) Project

Preface

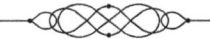

"We are now witnessing a natural experiment in the hospice market. Private equity firms seeing huge profits in buying hospice programs that are providing care for the most vulnerable persons and their families at a sentinel, often tragic time."

Joan M. Teno, MD, MS. Hospice Medical Director

SURVIVING HOSPICE: A CHAPLAIN'S JOURNEY INTO THE BUSINESS OF *Dying* is an eye-opening memoir about the extent to which commercial greed has invaded the hospice space. I include insider knowledge that the bad actors in the corporate hospice industry don't want patients, their families, employees, or the general public to know.

My book examines that "natural experiment" which was the infusion of professional investors into the end-of-life medical market which began in earnest in the early twenty-first century. When investor-owned hospice companies and stockholders position their financial interests ahead of the needs of patients, bad things happen. My account chronicles those *bad things* starting in 2012 when I worked for a Midwestern for-profit hospice chain as one of their chaplains.

My research-driven narrative evolved into a search for the crossroad when hospice care veered from the singular purpose of providing specialized care for the dying by linking pain and symptom control with compassion into a financial machine for cultivating wealth.

The original hospice model was a grass-roots movement once dominated by community and religious organizations; it was designed by physician Dame Cicely Saunders in England in 1963. What is hospice? A type of health care that focuses on the palliation of a terminally ill patient's pain and symptoms and attends to their emotional and spiritual needs at the end of life; or, as Senator Edward Kennedy said about its possibilities in 1978, "Hospice is many things . . . But most of all, hospice is the humanization of our health care system."

My book advances the knowledge about the hospice industry and accentuates the expansion of investor-owned hospice care since the ground-breaking work by journalists Sheila Himmel and Fran Smith in 2013. What I found is that the skyrocketing growth of the hospice market is not always centered on a benevolent embrace of the aging community and "the humanization of our health care system," but about a shrewd system of marketing predicated on profiteering and therefore, the exploitation of the dying.

I address this issue because the US hospice market has exploded with net revenues of $34.5 billion in 2022. Between 2011 and 2019, 72 percent of Medicare-certified hospices that were acquired by private equity and publicly-traded corporations were nonprofit.

Fortunately, for the genesis of this book, I accepted a job at the wrong place, but at the right time. It was the wrong place because approximately eighteen months into my employment our once trustworthy and mission-driven hospice care mysteriously deteriorated, and our office became a tense and stressful place to work. The palliative care and work environment slipped into something far less than what I was promised when I signed on the dotted line in 2010.

I believe that internal conflicts in a hospice workplace can occur when the primary interests of patients are incompatible with those of the owners and investors. I didn't know anything about the designations that labeled hospice companies as nonprofit or for-profit when I was searching for a job, and I had no idea about how to discern the quality of a hospice business or its subsequent care based on its economic structure.

Corporations that own hospice agencies are morally obligated to create a win/win situation for both patients and their businesses, but many do not. So, I highlight where to locate public data on the many companies that have not maintained that crucial balance.

My hospice employment transpired at the right time because I had unknowingly attained an advantageous platform from inside the company to witness negligence and unethical behavior. As time wore on, I realized the significance of my circumstances and the documentation I had in my possession. However, I had no idea of the consequences of the timing or how it would affect the next phase of my life.

After I left the company in 2014, it was important for me to take a partial hiatus from my official retirement to find out what happened at my company. During my research, I discovered that too many huge for-profit companies had misappropriated the Medicare and Medicaid Hospice Benefit and turned dying into a business commodity. Many hospice corporations have appropriate respect for their dying patients, but many do not. Hospice patients should never be treated like a *product* in a business portfolio.

In late 2022, *ProPublica* and *The New Yorker* co-published a report describing "how a visionary movement that provided dignity for the dying [hospice] has become a *plaything* for profiteers." I saw firsthand how our patients and staff came to be treated as puppets to generate immense profits.

Like puppets, we often felt that we were treated like objects. Puppets are a metaphor for those controlled by a more powerful person or group. Our worth was often measured by our level of compliance in maintaining a low overhead to sustain a healthy profit margin; no matter the cost to patients and families. The company had adopted a detached attitude.

So, after witnessing the escalation of harm to patients and the impudence toward staff at my company, Hospice Advantage, I could no longer sit shotgun. My silence felt complicit. Two years after my resignation, headlines across the country started to scream of the dereliction of duty toward patients that were in the custody of corporate-owned and publicly-traded hospice companies.

At the same time, experts at the National Institute On Aging (NIA) publicly speculated on a correlation between harm to patients, families, and staff, and the billions of dollars pumped into the procurement of American hospice companies.

Upon reading these frightening, but inevitable, bulletins, I knew I had something to contribute to that collective discussion. My book is the first on the market to corroborate the connection between private equity involvement in hospice and *harm to patients*. It was important for me to suspend the endless speculation with the truth of the matter. Also, through my research and years of volunteerism as a hospice consumer advocate, I demonstrate that my negative experience with our company was not an anomaly.

Two of my goals when I began this project six years ago were to help protect the image of the hospice benefit, and to uplift the *good actors* in the hospice industry, both nonprofit and for-profit.

There are many ways that readers can benefit from how I structured this book. In part one, the memoir section, you will learn how pastoral counseling and spiritual direction help terminally ill and dying patients. This section will also be useful for those studying to minister to the dying and for people who want to prepare for a good dying experience.

In part two, I provide an uplifting resource for consumers on how to find a trustworthy hospice company, whether it's nonprofit or for-profit. Incidentally, this section contains the only such guide on the market.

Finally, in part three, I address professionals associated with the hospice industry: hospice trade organizations, owners, lawmakers, insurance providers, professional investors, senior health-care providers, lawyers, hospice clinicians, and journalists.

You can purchase this book for the how-to guide to gain insight into finding a competent provider; to understand both the beauty and the grim reality of my pastoral work for the dying under the duress of owner avarice, and insight into the legislative, political, and economic aspects of the current hospice landscape.

However, it will be more meaningful if you read it in order. I hope the investigative sections of this book will give you the information you need to make a wise choice with end-of-life care.

Introduction

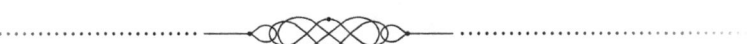

There are so many good hospice companies—both non-profit and in the for-profit sector (which is 80 percent of the hospice market). But while no medical care or economic structure is perfect, families must be apprised of the sobering fact that not all hospice companies are equal. My father cautioned me that if you want to know the goals behind any business, question the fundamental motivation for their establishment. The mission of a for-profit medical company that purchases hospices should be to maintain an equitable balance between uplifting humanity and responsible business ownership.

My intent in these chapters is to showcase both incompetent hospice practices and professional, successful hospice models. Successful, not in terms of a huge return on an investment, the acquisitions and mergers of hundreds of smaller hospices to profit from economies of scale, or the final masterstroke of buying and selling quickly (a three-year turnover rate is the norm) to achieve lucrative profits.

Truly, the definition of success for a hospice provider is the maintenance of a reputable and consistent clinical practice that administers the best medical resources for symptom control and timely pain management for a good quality of life until death.

This memoir is written through the lens of a chaplain and so it is primarily about the spiritual, religious, and emotional end-of-life stories of five people who suffered under the self-serving policies of my hospice company. Through poignant and often humorous stories, I expose the unethical practices and ignoble culture of my former company.

So much of the theology, spiritual perspectives, and religious knowledge that informed my pastoral counseling as a hospice chaplain originated with my spiritual director, Franciscan nun Jeannine Weidner; course work for my graduate theology degree at Cardinal Stritch University with Sister Coletta Dunn, and the CPE certification program and its director Father JoJo Orosa at St. Camillus Life Plan Community. Also, my own values and theology align closely with the prophetic and scriptural teachings by Franciscan priest Richard Rohr.

I selected the quotations that introduce each chapter to provide a concise description of my beliefs about each subsequent narrative.

The Health Insurance Accountability Act (HIPAA) sets standards and regulations to protect health information and patient privacy. To maintain these standards in my narrative, I have reviewed the guidelines for confidentiality in the HIPPA. I was not able to locate the families of my deceased patients, so I fictionalized identifying information. The stories I relate are a composite of my actual experiences ministering to patients and families over the course of my hospice internship and clinical career.

Incidentally, it's important to understand that chaplains are trained to retain patient information and to archive it for documentation. We learn to write verbatims (word-for-word notes) during hospice visits to accurately record patient comments and the type of counseling provided at each appointment. I also learned to keep extensive notes on my patients to accurately reflect their lives to deliver heartfelt eulogies at their funerals.

My former company no longer exists; it has been flipped, flopped, stripped, sanitized, percolated, and buried under many equity-firm acquisitions and mergers. The names of the financial players in this narrative are the actual firms involved. The information about their goals and financial transactions in the hospice industry came from their own websites and substantiated news articles.

Also, much of the data for my narrative in the chapters titled, "A Gold Mine" and "Dying For Dollars" was written by journalists Sheila Himmel and Fran Smith in their book, *Changing The Way We Die*. Ms. Himmel granted written permission to utilize the specific research in chapter twelve for my account.

PART ONE

Spiritual Stories of Crossing the Threshold

Going Back

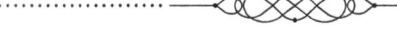

"Just when I think I understand how to walk through the door, it shrinks or the locks change."

Lewis Carroll, Alice in Wonderland

My curiosity piqued, I made a split-second decision, veered off the freeway, and turned north toward my former workplace, just to see what I might find. I navigated the familiar potholes and crossed the double row of railroad tracks.

So many memories flooded my thoughts as I neared my destination. Over the course of a few years, unscrupulous decisions made by our corporate headquarters began to shape the policies and procedures of this local hospice agency.

Even after I left the company, those distressing memories persisted. At first, only threadlike tendrils of bad experiences clung to my soul. So fragile, they lay in the shallow—unobtrusive and tight-lipped. Weightless, but evocative, just the same. The distance between the negative experiences and my retirement was a relatively comfortable yoke upon my shoulders.

Unexpectedly, the latent memories found a way to unfurl and flourish—pushing forward toward the light of day like the truth of a thing—probing for oxygen, acceptance, purpose, and respect. Old, familiar voices surfaced and maneuvered their way into my daytime awareness—like the late-term infant pushing and kicking the muscular inner layer of the uterus—frantic to be released. Relentless in her pursuit to be known. Or at least, to be considered. Was it the snippets of unfavorable hospice headlines that suddenly appeared sporadically across the country that stirred my sleep? I had managed to ignore these furtive messages for months.

Poet Maya Angelou once mused, "There is no greater agony than bearing an untold story inside you." Yes, I suppose that is true. But I didn't really believe that I had a story. All I had were questions with no answers. The unfortunate consequences of unethical decision-making. A pit in my stomach. Flimsy assumptions and a jumble of justifiable anger. Not the stuff of credible storytelling. How would I fill in the blanks and connect the dots? It was complicated. I was a music educator, a religion teacher, and a chaplain; not a seasoned writer. And in the end, would it even matter? After all, time often softens the remnants of harm and seems to sweep them out of view. We easily forget.

From a block away, I glimpsed the faded turquoise lettering on a hillside billboard that towered above our offices. Drivers saw the advertisement for miles in all directions. Hospice Advantage: *"Care, Comfort, and Compassion for the Whole Family."* I felt a wave of apprehension as I caught sight of the logo. The clinical staff had been reduced to a skeletal team of loyalists by 2014, but I was not one of them. The vestiges of my loyalty had swirled down the sewer after their high-pressure tactics to swap our health insurance, so I had refused the company's offer of a per diem chaplain role.

As I turned down the asphalt driveway, a vacant parking lot greeted me. This was a surprise for a mid-afternoon on a weekday. I idled the car for a few minutes to survey my surroundings, and then I stepped out onto the abandoned property. Flakes of snow dusted the air, and I fumbled for the buttons on my coat. Relief washed over me as a "for sale" sign captured my interest. I hadn't really planned to run into anyone; I wasn't even sure why I was there.

Our hospice agency had occupied the lower level of a two-story building. Weeds poked through the white landscape stone around the perimeter, and the grassy areas could no longer be described as a bona fide lawn. A few blinds hung haphazardly enough to allow me to peer inside. The large room was empty, except for an array of metal filing cabinets lining a long wall, some with drawers left wide open. Cardboard boxes crammed with empty turquoise binders and piles of shredded documents awaited disposal. I walked around to the main entrance. Heavy, looping chain shackled the handles of both glass doors like the manacled wrists of a defiant prisoner awaiting a verdict.

We had been one of the most professional providers in southeastern Wisconsin. I strode around to the east side of the building and peeked into the conference room, remembering one of many challenging cases. In my third week on the job, I arrived at 7:30 a.m. and bumped into one of our medical directors at the front desk. The first words out of his mouth were, "I'm glad I'm not in your shoes right now." He cocked his head toward the conference room. "The rest of your team is waiting for you."

Good morning to you too, Dr. Patel.

Immediately, my mind raced from A to Z. Did I do something wrong already? I'm just getting my feet wet here. Surveying the lay of the land. Figuring out what's what and who's who and where the supplies were located.

My pulse quickened as I rounded the corner and stopped just short of the conference-room door to find members of my interdisciplinary team gathered inside around the oblong table, drinking black coffee. No doughnuts or creamer in sight. No idle chatter, just heads huddled. When I entered the room, four somber faces turned to me in unison. Dread washed over me; it was the feeling one experiences walking alone down a deserted alley in the wrong part of town in the dark.

As I pulled up a chair, Sandy, the registered nurse announced, "A chaplain is the most qualified person for this situation. You should go first."

They all nodded.

What situation? Where? *I'm the rookie here, remember?* But I understood. I was that golden canary lowered into a pitch-black shaft of coal to warn the foreman pacing up top if poisonous gas awaited. Miners often hauled up a filthy, dead-as-a-doornail canary. Okay. Fine. The chaplain would go first. It's amazing what could be uncovered if a person (or a bird) went deep enough.

Each hospice patient is assigned an interdisciplinary team. The RN is the manager of the team and directs the care. I sat down with my team to absorb the terrible news that spilled from their elbow-to-elbow meeting. My earlier panic had dissipated at the disclosure, though an admonishment would've been better than the reality that awaited me.

The only son of one of my dying patients had been killed in a car accident, the victim of a drunken driver. He was twenty-four. His father Don, fifty-two, had been diagnosed with pancreatic cancer and had only weeks to live. They needed someone at the house to support Carla, the wife and mother. That "someone" was me. She was alone that morning until her daughter returned from Michigan. The RN might've sent our social worker, but the family was religious.

That tragic event tested every ounce of my training. I rearranged my schedule for the morning and set my GPS for 101 Clondike Street. I'd seen Carla at the skilled-nursing facility where her husband was on our hospice service, but I had never visited their home. When I arrived at the modest neighborhood in an older section of town, Carla was dragging an overstuffed container of garbage out of the garage. I parked on the tree-lined street in front of their Cape Cod-style house.

Taking a few deep breaths, I gathered my belongings and approached her. She continued to haul the blue container toward the street, her expression dour. I lowered my briefcase of bereavement materials and paperwork to the lawn and coaxed the bin of recyclables from her grasp. She turned back for more. We heaved a few more overflowing containers of old newspapers and cans on top of the collection she had already deposited at the curb. In silence.

Unfortunately, weekly routines resume even in the face of catastrophe. When our world collapses, we cling to habits and rote tasks that give us a sense of normalcy and a measure of control. Self-protection, I called it. After all, it was a Thursday and time for the weekly garbage and recycling collection. Dumping refuse was like death, suffering, taxes, and love—there was no getting around it. And decluttering created space for something new. After all, wasn't it like a spiritual act, inevitable and imperative?

But letting go of loved ones was an entirely different matter.

I joined her in the kitchen and engulfed her in a hug. I looked into her blue-eyed saucers of sorrow and then down at the photos of Michael scattered across the table: snapshots of his baptism, birthdays, Christmas, prom, and in his Marine uniform. In a few short weeks, she would stare at another batch of memories. Her wedding, honeymoon, family gatherings, and the births of children.

Dear God.

Carla offered me a cigarette. I didn't smoke, but I accepted it anyway. It was a bonding opportunity. She leaned in to offer me a light. I barely knew what to do with it. But we were spiritual comrades now, and we smoked our way through thickets of grief that morning. We chain-smoked her menthols and washed down a plate of cinnamon doughnuts with cup after cup of jet-black coffee. I usually drank a moderate amount of coffee with a lot of cream and sugar, but this tragic occasion begged for something stronger. My stomach was roiling.

I felt out of sorts with the unfamiliar fare, but it did contain four of the five major food groups: caffeine, nicotine, sugar, and fat. Adequate fare for the planning of a funeral. Artificial comfort soothed us for now. I let her talk and talk and talk. And weep. We prayed. She asked questions. I offered spiritual resources, scripture passages, grief support groups, and pastoral wisdom. I left space for silence. She slammed her fist on the table.

We decided not to tell her husband . . . not just yet. It might hasten his own earthly departure, and she desperately needed every ounce of what was left of him. She pondered whether to wait and hold both funerals together—it's amazing how shock-induced numbness lingers long enough to help survivors get through the devastating details of planning even one funeral.

When a neighbor dropped by, I rose to leave and headed toward my next patient. Before I left, I handed Carla two white tapers to place in her front window during the upcoming holidays. When lit, these candles would signify the ongoing light of her departed loved ones in the next world. We hugged, and I shut the door on her misery.

I sat in my car at the curb surveying the neat, orderly lawns of this neighborhood and resetting my GPS for my next patient. No one walking by would suspect the chaos that had just descended upon this house.

That husband and wife had been my true initiation into hospice work. I had handled the task set before me that morning. Barely. That day, I realized I was in an honorable profession. A true vocation. It felt right.

While I mused about the past, the snowfall had thickened. Shivering, I backed away from the window and Carla faded from view. The vignette was like an impressionistic painting: a hazy mirage of a lonely woman at the height of suffering.

I had left my car in my former parking spot, the third row from the building, even though the lot was empty. Habits did die hard. I drove away for the final time. However, I had a phone call to make.

The First Year

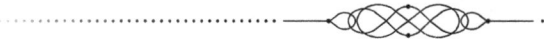

"To give real service, you must add something which cannot be bought or measured with money, and that is sincerity and integrity."

Douglas Adams, English author

On August 1, 2010, I signed a full-time contract with a thriving hospice practice. This vocation was my third career. Before that, I had spent twenty years in education. I managed two high school vocal music programs, and then I obtained a graduate degree in religious studies, and taught church history and morality courses at the secondary level.

My professional tools changed from musical scores, scripts, and librettos to religious textbooks, holy water, and bibles. My hands, once trained for playing the piano and conducting became instruments to create classroom lectures, church history maps, and video presentations on medieval saints. And as a chaplain, to bless foreheads, anoint broken bodies, and distribute Communion.

My career path meandered with uncertainty at times, but guideposts seemed to appear just when I really needed them. The sign that sparked my interest in a religious ministry was a definition of "chaplaincy" that I stumbled upon in a religious studies class. "Chaplains help patients [and themselves] find the communal meaning and significance of the suffering of all life so as not to retreat into their small worlds in the misguided quest for personal safety and sanity."

"Misguided quest?" Personal safety and a measure of sanity sounded sensible to me. That provocative definition intrigued me; and yet, I felt intimidated by the implications of its tall order. It jarred something deep within me like when I visited the formidable Berlin Wall in 1973.

After serious consideration, I searched for information on the profession of chaplaincy. When I joined the hospice agency, it was one of the dozens providing care in southeastern Wisconsin. All ten offices in the spacious, first-floor agency bustled with end-of-life expertise. With ninety patients registered and enrollment climbing, we were a middle-sized company attending to the pain and symptoms of terminally ill patients.

Hospice care revolves around the idea that suffering at the end of life stems not only from the physical ravages of the disease but also from the emotional component and social issues surrounding care. Our teams did a wonderful job helping people die well. It was so rewarding to work at Hospice Advantage (HA) in those ensuing months.

Our company was founded in 2004, during the spread of hospice commercial ventures across the country. HA was headquartered in Bay City, Michigan, and was one of the nation's largest privately-held hospice organizations. It owned fifty-six agencies sprinkled across eleven states throughout the Midwest and South. While the bulk of our patients lived in skilled-nursing homes, we also offered a home-based, health-care division when I came on board.

We had a small staff: two medical directors, an administrator, an office manager, six certified hospice RNs, two social workers, six certified nursing assistants, a volunteer coordinator, a bereavement counselor, an on-call third-shift RN, and three full-time marketing representatives. We had a balanced patient-staff ratio and a reputation for distinction.

We wore bright turquoise smocks and scrubs that announced our brand and presence in the twenty nursing homes where we were contracted to work. We were walking billboards for Hospice Advantage. Our intricate logo, a variation of the Trinity spiral, was derived from an ancient Celtic icon that symbolized the interplay between birth, death, and rebirth. That logo represented the spiritual maturity that human beings gained from the trials of aging, managing life, and facing mortality. A company that innately understood the sanctity of the life-and-death cycle was one I wanted to work for.

The turquoise emblem adorned every speck of marketing merchandise, medical apparatus, and corporate stationery. The color turquoise is associated with spiritual grounding, tranquility, and emotional balance. Those characteristics were outcomes that chaplains strived to achieve with dying patients, their families, and themselves.

I always thought that our company name was atypical: Hospice Advantage. Most hospice companies branded their business to end-of-life metaphors such as horizon, seasons, legacy, and rainbows. I assumed the rationale behind our name was that the company had an "advantage" in service compared to other providers; that we had the upper hand and the leading edge for bestowing expert care. Hospice consumers could place their confidence in us.

Our motto, "Care, Comfort, and Compassion for the Whole Family," conveyed the crucial needs of the dying. We had aligned our mission with those values. All hospice companies should manage their businesses in such a way that their mission and bottom line translate into social and moral responsibility.

Looking back, I realized that I had embarked on a career in hospice at a time when the US hospice industry had experienced considerable turbulence in the previous decade from changes in ownership, growth, and the shift to for-profit status.

During my first months on the job, I quickly learned that competition between companies could be cutthroat, and even minor clinical mistakes could get any company yanked from a facility. Most of my dying patients resided in nursing homes. Marketers, under heavy pressure to increase patient enrollment in early 2012, often consulted our interdisciplinary team to discuss strategies that might enhance goodwill at a facility. At one point, it seemed as if we were more obligated to our marketing personnel than to our RN case managers.

As we sat bedside, our reps wandered through hallways schmoozing facility staff and managers with baked goods, bed-and-bath products, and catered lunches. Marketers dispensed cheer along with chocolate bars to employee lounges. I found it curious that our clinical staff was required to spend precious hours hobnobbing with facility administrators over layers of Italian pasta and garlic bread. After all, in skilled nursing facilities, sick patients turned into dying patients, and dying patients needed hospice.

Walking a competitive tightrope with ten or more hospice companies often translates into promises and compromises. If the blue-garbed hospice company pledged weighted lap blankets, we countered with audio headsets programmed to the serenity of lapping waves. If the purple-outfitted providers in the next wing offered pet therapy, we proposed music therapy even though I was a music educator and not a music therapist. It was a clever game of chess to outmaneuver our competitors. I had no idea of the scope of it.

Today, many nursing homes find it easier to initiate their own hospice services than to contract with outsiders. They have more control, and they deal with less complaints.

Meanwhile, back in windowless conference rooms, visiting corporate executives were hunkered down conceiving recruitment schemes to increase the number of patients. They flew to all sixty agencies, rallying the employees with contests offering gift certificates, meals, and bonuses. One colleague won the $2,000 grand prize for increasing our census by five patients.

We hired expensive marketers and purchased shiny white sedans with our company name emblazoned across their doors. Generous bonuses were awarded to our sales staff and regional managers for increasing our census. One of my colleagues in the marketing division said sales representatives were promised an additional $200 per client after their patient quota for the month had been met. Our practice was booming.

Love and Delight

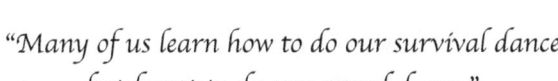

*"Many of us learn how to do our survival dance
but forget to do our sacred dance."*

Bill Plotkin, psychologist and author

MY INAUGURATION INTO THE HOSPICE MOVEMENT BEGAN at the bedside of my dying mother. She was the reason I was inspired to investigate the profession in 2009. She experienced a "good death" as hospice professionals liked to coin an optimal dying experience, so I placed her story first. Consumers need to understand what a good dying experience looks like so that they can be discerning when shopping for a hospice. Unfortunately, not all hospices give the same level of care.

Actually, my mother's final hours were better than good. Claire spent her last hours in a nonprofit, inpatient hospice residence in comfort and peaceful. I was so inspired by her serene and sacred dying process that it sparked a new career interest, and that's when I researched the requirements for hospice chaplaincy.

I had a degree in religious studies, so it wasn't a huge leap to study for chaplaincy. A few months after Mom's funeral, I applied to the program. By the next June, I had started clinical pastoral education (CPE) and the formation for chaplaincy. CPE is essentially a hands-on program focused on exposing students to vulnerable and often intense spiritual care situations in hospitals and nursing homes to help them become more effective pastoral ministers. I wanted to provide for others what my own mother had experienced during her final hours.

Her final day on this good earth had dawned cloudy and cold. I remember how restless she seemed, more agitated than usual. Lying next to her, I was aware of costumed trick-or-treaters prancing up and down the hallway past our door. We looked out the window across the golden meadow, cuddling amidst tangled sheets, and wisps of her silky hair brushed against my cheek.

The deathbed vigil had lingered for days, and we had finally taken up shifts. My brothers and their children had driven back to their homes to catch up on work and take a short reprieve. My elderly father was exhausted, so I sent him home to rest.

I pointed to the field swallow standing guard over her young brood. Mom whistled their song. Even in her weakened condition, she could mimic any bird call. I smiled at her melodic trill though tears prickled beneath my lashes. A sob caught in my throat, threatening our tranquility, and I fought to smother the eruption of sorrow. I didn't want to upset her.

With feeble effort, she tried to tighten my already firm grip around her. She had shuffled around for months with fallen arches and stooped shoulders. Bunions rubbed raw at the edges of her woolen slippers—slippers so tattered, they barely contained her nylon-enshrouded feet. Dementia had devastated her brain, and cancer ravaged her one drooping breast and had also sprouted in her ovaries. But in my mind, she remained as stately as the silver birch that shaded the woodland stream out back.

As the hours wore on, her breathing became labored. I imagined her soul yearning for freedom from its earthly womb with a looming instinct that the confining space was only meant to be temporary and that a mysterious, magnificent world lay within reach. She shivered beneath the quilt. "What would I have done without you?" Those would be her last words.

The dying process progressed, and I sensed her increasing unease. Her fear was palpable. My inclination to hinder its headway was no match for her soul's resolve to be released. I wanted to continue hovering and doting over her, but a mother won't surrender easily with a daughter clinging to her hip.

I relaxed my grip on her life with the hushed singing of a Shaker lullaby she once sang to me. *"'Tis the gift to be simple, 'tis the gift to be free, 'tis the gift to come down where you ought to be, and when you find yourself in the place just right, you'll be in the valley of love and delight."* My voice stumbled over the refrain. *"When true simplicity is . . . gained . . . to bow and to bend . . ."* I couldn't finish.

I gently pried her from me and positioned another pillow beneath her head. Settling into a chair, I clasped her hand and watched the hours of dusk disappear. Sunlight receded, and soon shadows danced across the floor to the strains of Schubert's "Ave Maria." The room filled with the aroma of lavender as I anointed her hands and feet. Prayerfully, I nudged Mom toward the "valley of love and delight" resplendent with her favorite purple petunias, choirs of angelic singing, and wholeness.

My eighty-year-old mother had become unresponsive, but the staff claimed she could still hear me.

"I love you, Mom," I announced with conviction, testing their assumption.

Her eyelids quivered.

Midnight passed, and the nursing schedule shifted. Concerned staff members had come and gone with morphine and other antidotes for discomfort. After standing to stretch, I crossed the room to take in the view. Shards of starlight graced the garden, a labyrinth of sleepy flowers and boxy hedge where lightning bugs darted and flashed, and chalky-white angelic sculptures and stone benches glowed in ghostly repose.

I turned to her wedding portrait that my father had placed on the table. Maybe he had wanted to focus on the memories of her as a voluptuous twenty-four-year-old beauty instead of the unrecognizable form lying before me—all wrinkles and shriveled husk.

In the sepia photograph, dated 1952, her dark, shoulder-length curls were framed by a modest chiffon veil secured to a simple tiara braided with lilies of the valley. I looked nothing like her: she was olive-skinned and French. I was blonde and fair with my German and Norwegian genes dominating any French bloodlines. While I resembled my father's family, a great deal about me came from her.

I remember how long that night seemed to linger. I filled its solitude with the flickering of candlelight and the calming recitation of the rosary. Any mantra would've sufficed. All those hours sitting at death's door propelled miles of memories forward until they dribbled to nothing. Loneliness and despair overwhelmed me as the painful truth settled in—our memory-making was nearly finished.

Searching the shadows, I wondered if our ancestors were present, waiting to escort Mom home. I fantasized that her four sisters, my favorite aunts, were fussing over us like a clutch of chubby hens bobbing and clucking. That consoling reverie was an unexpected respite and made me lose track of Mom's decline.

For the final three hours, her breathing would cease for stretches of forty-five seconds. I would think death was at hand, only to see her snatch erratic gulps of stale air to prolong the vigil. Her skeletal shoulders heaved inward with each inhalation, and the breathy discharge gurgled and crackled its way into the room. The nurse insisted she didn't feel any pain. But I was only partly comforted. My mother should've passed on by now, the staff had told me. But she was always a fighter, that one. Stubborn.

"Mom, it's okay to let go. We'll be all right. You can help us from heaven."

Maybe she just needed to maintain a sense of dignity and privacy and wanted to die on her own terms. Alone. She would never want me to anguish watching her labor for oxygen. The staff had encouraged me to go home and get some sleep that night, but I couldn't leave her.

Her apnea was increasing, so I began the tedious count once again. By the time I reached fifty-five seconds, my heart was racing. I waited . . . and waited . . . and waited. But she did not struggle to inhale. Finding no pulse, I withdrew my trembling hand.

I still needed her . . . I wasn't ready.

"Mom, don't leave me," I wailed into the night.

I got up and paced.

Staring out into the gardens with my back to her, I marveled at how my "bird whistler" no longer existed in this world. I dared to turn and confront her fate. She lay with such serenity, her eyes like cumbersome drapes that were partially drawn. Her features were lackluster and ashen; her jaw hung loosely. How quickly death had ferried her away. Wracking sobs took hold of my gut, and I could no longer restrain a torrent of tears. I slid to my knees beside her.

A good mother should never die. A good mother should never die. A good mother should never, ever die.

I tried to convince myself that she was simply standing just beyond my vision. Watching me.

Finally, after long minutes of anguish, a serenity washed over the room. I sensed the crowning of her soul, as if lilies and kindness, lilacs and grace had gushed forth with her essence. Her face, a vision of peace and pride, as her labor ended. Triumphant even. I planted a kiss on her warm, familiar cheek.

Cradling her still body in my arms, I memorized her scent—hair hinting of roses, skin oozing musk and lavender. From now on, her final scent would be my new cologne. I laid her down on the bed and gathered the knobby quilt to her chin, tucking it in tight, as if bolting a door against the chill of winter.

As I glanced out at the sky, the first blush of dawn greeted me. On that fresh morn, she would not rise with the lark. I should've awakened my father, but I wanted her to myself a few moments longer. It was selfish, I know. But she was my mother . . . my only sister . . . my friend. But looking back, I might've been forestalling my father's arrival to spare him this scene. I'd only seen him cry once in my life, at the gravesite of his father. It was unsettling. I didn't know if I could bear his suffering now, too.

After grabbing my makeup bag, I reapplied my ruby-shaded lipstick and firmly planted a final kiss. A bold last gesture. But I didn't care. There, for all to witness, was the mark of affection emblazoned on her forehead, like the Hindu Bindi, the feminine embellishment that signified the achievement of one's earthly purpose. She had birthed her soul in this room. She left a sliver of her soul with me, and I bathed in its wholeness and holiness.

I searched her face. Her eyes were vacant. I no longer possessed an earthly mother. After calling my father and breaking the news, I lowered her lids and placed a wad of cloths beneath her chin to hold it in place. When my father arrived, he would only see that she slept peacefully. As I watched him escort the gurney out of the building to the waiting hearse, he fumbled to locate her hand, or perhaps the curve of a hip, sheathed within the black body bag. He stood erect just like the morning he offered his arm to usher her out of the church, his bride adorned in joy and veiled in white tulle.

I remembered the refrain of the Shaker song my mother had sung to me as a child: *When true simplicity is gained, to bow and to bend, we shall not be ashamed. To turn, turn, will be our delight, till by turning, turning we come round right.*

The term "turning" has Latin roots in the word *conversio,* and the song symbolizes how the "turning" and "bending" of the soul throughout life correlates with a conversion of the heart. The inner spiritual work of "turning" and "bending" is emotionally painful, but necessary. The theology was too advanced for a five-year-old, but my mother and I had danced to the tidy rhythms in the garden as the Shakers had in their religious services. She had undergone the "turning" process and had "come 'round right." Her earthly purpose was complete.

I left the hospice residence and stumbled out into life without my bird whistler. I'll always remember that moment, how unsteady and disoriented I felt. Suddenly, a burst of energy rushed through me, and I shivered. I recognized my mother's final, glancing touch. I felt her soul take flight, effortless and robust once again. On course and confident. "To a place just right."

I gazed into the flaxen meadow, where birds gathered and fluttered and sang. And from somewhere, just beyond the stars, I heard her mimic their song.

On-Call

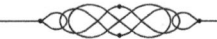

*"You matter until the end of your life. We will do
all that we can to help you die peacefully."*
Dame Cicely Saunders, founder of the modern hospice movement

A SLICE OF DAWN PENETRATED THE BROKEN SLAT ON THE blind and interrupted my satisfying sleep. It was a dreary morning—windy and wet. I hated waking early on a weekend, especially if it was a plan wrecker type of day. Sunday was meant to be a day for rest, after all. My husband, Mark, was sleeping beside me, his muscular six-foot-two frame stretched from headboard to footboard, wisps of air from his CPAP machine pulsating with each inhalation. That nightly white noise was as soothing as waves lapping at the shore.

A sudden gust of wind whipped at the pane, rattling the glass.

I slipped from the chilly room to make breakfast and filled animal bowls as the heavy residue from a night of sound sleep receded. When I returned to the warm flannel sheets, I recalled a warning by Rumi, one of my favorite writers and a thirteenth-century Sufi mystic: "The breeze at dawn has secrets to tell you. Do not go back to sleep."

Rumi, the breeze has already revealed itself but has not unleashed its mysterious message, and the sun has already reached the top of the horizon. So . . . you're late. Spit it out. I'm not big on secrets anyway—whatever it was you came to say, say it. And by the way, how does the "breeze at dawn" go about unveiling a subliminal message?

Rumi's poem, "The Breeze at Dawn" reminds us to step into the day, into wakefulness. "Wherever we find ourselves, there are new opportunities." This is a poem not only about the morning hours, but about any transition from night to day, or life to death. It suggests that the movement is not only going in one direction, but rather "back and forth" between different states. If we get underneath the surface, listen deeply to the secrets of the breeze, and ask for what we really want, a new level of awakening is available.

Well, I guess I was up for the day. I'd been reduced to mumbling to dead poets. There is a society for that, I think. Mostly, I needed a break from hospice work—somewhere warm.

I settled against a mound of feather pillows, the casings edged with scallops of French lace from the region of Alsace-Lorraine. The lace had been handed down from my great-great-grandmother. I envisioned her reaching through generations of female ancestors to enfold me in maternal affection. As I looked over the contingent of critters who were vying for jurisdiction over our king-sized bed—a tangle of paws and limbs, tails, and toes—I absorbed the pleasure of that domestic tableau through every pore.

I wedged a wicker tray between us, a not-so-subtle hint for Mark to wake up. As I picked at the coffee cake and warmed my spirit with sips of chai, my cell buzzed. Mark stirred at the piercing tone. I retreated to another room hoping it was the transplant coordinator from the University of Wisconsin Hospitals. Mark had suffered a massive heart attack the previous Valentine's Day near Prairie du Chien, Wisconsin, and had been airlifted to Gundersen Lutheran Hospital in La Crosse for triple-bypass surgery and the placement of a defibrillator. Heart attacks should be outlawed on Valentine's Day.

He had been accepted into the transplant program in Madison. We were instructed to stay close to home, which meant not venturing more than four hours from our front stoop in case an organ became available. I was disappointed to hear the serious voice of our weekend-shift RN.

"One of your new patients is declining. John Schwartz."

"Yes. Okay. Got it. Prognosis?" I grabbed a notepad as she continued.

"Not good. A few days, maybe a week—if he's lucky." I told her I'd be on my way. John, who was grappling with end-stage liver cancer, also had schizophrenia. Or perhaps it might be more accurate to say that John grappled with schizophrenia and also had liver cancer; either way, the combination of both afflictions doubled his suffering and challenged my expertise. It was a tough case.

How did I help a patient embrace the inner presence of Divine Light when that gentle stirring competed with the dark, brutal voices rooted in a serious mental disorder? How did I manage it?

When I got off the phone and returned to the bedroom, Mark was devouring a bagel smothered in cream cheese. Ruddy indentations imprinted by the rigid rim of the CPAP mask crisscrossed his face, chin to cheekbones, the cosmetic cost of healthy sleep and no snoring. I smiled.

"What?" he deadpanned.

He always looked a bit ragged in the morning with those trails embedded in his face. I crawled back into bed. Some people had bad hair days, but Mark didn't have much hair. Bad face days were his scourge. We all had something.

"Do people at work even take you seriously before ten?" I teased.

He snorted affectionately in my ear. My smile slid.

"Let me guess. You just forfeited your day off," he said.

I was scheduled for on-call hours that weekend, but I hadn't planned to work based on the medical notes from the Saturday night, second-shift RN. Everyone was stable then, which meant nothing, of course, in the medical business. The week had been taxing, so I'd counted on the weekend to unwind and have something besides death to occupy my thoughts. It's not that I didn't enjoy my profession. I just craved timely respites from its intense demands.

At times, I found it easier to address the spiritual and emotional issues of my dying patient than to navigate the complexities of their immediate family members. Families are complicated, and during the dying process unexpected issues arise. But in hospice, the patient and the family are considered one unit of care.

During the past week, I'd refereed arguments between the grieving adult children of one patient about *the will* and perceived favoritism and then listened to a wrenching bedside confession about marital infidelity from a man whose unsuspecting wife was on her way to the facility. And then, a well-meaning daughter fretted within earshot of her dying, devout Presbyterian mother on whether she had been born again and truly saved for eternal life. Most patients requested a chaplain to help sort through spiritual or religious matters. I received occasional help when patients had pastors. Many did not, including John.

Mark offered a plausible plan to placate my disappointment. "If you get home early enough, we can watch a movie. You'll need a double dose of a romantic comedy by the time you walk through the door. I'll order pizza." My smile crept back as he recited the details. Thin crust. Sausage. Mushroom. Onion. A bit of basil. With a side of ranch dressing. My favorite. *My man.*

"And a six-pack of Stella, please," I added.

I reached for my soul-mate, swiped at the remnant of cream cheese on his chin, and placed it on my tongue. Wrapping my leg around his thigh, I enjoyed his sweet kisses, and then I looked at the clock. Time was a taskmaster. I threw back the comforter and started for the bathroom, but he pulled me back for one final kiss.

On my final pass through the bedroom, I chuckled at the three furry squatters who had staked claims on my side of the bed: our sweet black Labrador, my daughter's Siamese prima-donna, and her gray tabby with a penchant for mischief. We were cat sitting. Three sets of inquisitive eyes—vivid brown, green, and gray—scrutinized my every move. I knew what the cats were thinking: *Don't let the door hit you on your way out.*

This nursing home was thirty minutes away in an under-resourced, inner-city neighborhood plagued by criminal activity. I usually took a colleague along, but no one was available that weekend. As I pulled into the parking lot, it relieved me to see deserted streets around the building. Apparently, the drug dealers had spent a late night on the town.

In some ways, this was my least favorite facility to visit because the building, along with its patients, had endured years of neglect. But maybe it was my favorite for the same reason; long lives filled with neglect had converted many of its ragged residents into premature saints. Medicaid facilities must admit everyone, so the wealthy and privileged went to die in the upscale facility across town. I often preferred ministering to Medicaid patients. Those folks were poor, vulnerable, and acclimated to living on the margins of life. Their humility made them insightful tutors and the best storytellers.

I'd always thought I'd die in a place of luxury, but I've reflected on my own dying process during hundreds of deathbed vigils. Maybe I'd like to be buried in a shroud of burlap, my corpse serving as compost for flowers, bees, butterflies, and trees in fields that pose as a park—void of towering grave markers but strewn with plenty of benches.

We might consider a cemetery as sacred as a theological library that harbors volumes of ancient primary sources, and musty manuscripts; a sanctuary of orderly spines to peruse and ponder in row after row of floor-to-ceiling shelves. When I meander through the irregular plots of disturbed earth, labelled with names and dates staked to final epitaphs, I realize how many unique stories there are to unearth. Bestsellers and debacles alike.

John

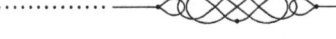

*"Let's take advantage of this exquisite time
while everything is broken down."*

Lee Blessing, playwright

WHEN I REACHED THE NURSE'S STATION, I GRABBED THE turquoise binder for John Adams Schwartz, age fifty-eight, and trudged to his room. His bed was on the far side of the double-occupancy space. Closer to the door, his groggy roommate sat at the edge of his bed. I smiled as I passed.

At first glance, John appeared unresponsive. But a slight rise and fall of his chest squelched my concern. For a minute. Then panic seized me. Perhaps it might've been better to stumble upon a warm corpse. I had never ministered to a dying person wrestling with schizophrenia.

Physicians were not the only professionals warned to *do no harm*. I attempted to leave a soul in better condition than I found it. The essence of a soul was sacred. Mystic Julian of Norwich often spoke of God "resting in the human soul." Therefore, do we do to God what we do to ourselves? Regardless, a minister must use caution when tampering with the divine presence. I tried not to inflict further harm upon my patient with an errant practice, a false doctrine, or off-the-cuff spiritual quackery. I have enough culpability for my own soul.

John's skin had a yellowish cast, and I detected the odor of necrotic tissue. I rarely experienced the sickeningly sweet odor of death on my patients, but after examining his file, I saw he had undergone a surgery that had not fully healed. *The poor fellow in Bed A.* Tugging on the privacy curtain, I gathered it around us.

Nausea rising to my throat, I removed a mask from my pocket and inserted a sponge soaked and dried in orange-infused oil to purify my cotton shield and neutralize the odor. Next, I arranged for a fan and a strong room deodorizer. *Poor John.* I gave the warped sash of the window a nudge upward, and the pent-up fetidity filtered through the screen. Hopefully, a swirl of crisp autumn air was awaiting its cue to rush forward and occupy what had been evicted. *Yes, Rumi—I'm sure the breeze responsible for "the secret message" is cooling its heels just outside our window.* Perhaps the secret messages were divine instructions on how to minister to a dying man with schizophrenia. I could only hope such wisdom was pending. The day was young.

Only ninety minutes earlier, I was engulfed in my husband's comforting arms beneath flannel sheets, inhaling the fragrance of Old Spice. The woodsy scent still clung to my skin. It wasn't too difficult to shepherd the dying during a typical forty-hour work week—dying became routine by Friday. But on a Sunday, when I was on call, I shuffled toward death.

I returned to the file for the "highlights" of John's life. *Birth:10-12-1953. Single male. Three siblings, all living. Parents, deceased. DX: clinical depression in early teens; paranoid schizophrenia diagnosed at 19. HS dropout. Behavioral-medicine inpatient/1970. Entered Oak Crest group home at 30. Criminal incidents X3. History of alcohol/drug use. Truancy. Religion: Protestant. Burial: Cremation.*

John was only middle-aged, but a life of "self-medication" to battle severe mental illness had taken its toll. Reading further, I saw the bold lettering: **Family is estranged.** This was a further concern, but not surprising. Schizophrenia was rough on the entire family. A recent addendum to the chart specified that our social worker had been awaiting more information from the group-home manager.

How sad to see fifty-eight years of a life crammed into such a concise and clinical biography. He was more than his illness. I checked the list of medications, relieved to see John was being treated with anti-psychotic drugs. That would make it easier to help him. Once I closed the file, I lowered the binder to the floor and dragged my chair closer.

"Mr. Schwartz, can you hear me?"

Without warning, a wide-eyed aide strutted through the drawn curtain—a boxy fan snug to her underarm—crashing headlong into our stillness like a bowling ball barreling down upon the ten unsuspecting pins. She located an outlet, set the dial on medium, and backed out of our death chamber in haste just as she had arrived—breathless and skittish. I couldn't blame her.

As I plugged in an aromatherapy diffuser that purified the air and dispensed essential oils, I chose eucalyptus for John. It had a delicate balsamic aroma that promoted serenity, emotional balance, and spiritual healing. We would all benefit by dabbing that essence on our pulse points each morning.

I wish I could've offered John a cup of chamomile tea sweetened with honey and a hug—an antidote a wife, mother, daughter, or close friend would've brought to the bed of a dying man. Searching the room for personal items that might give me insight into this mysterious man, I noticed a small wooden shelf containing assorted belongings: a framed photo of a horse tied to a fence; a blue and orange Mets cap; an album of *Sgt. Pepper's Lonely Hearts Club Band*; a tattered copy of *The Hobbit* that looked as if it had just emerged from a teenage boy's back pocket; and a family photograph propped against the paperback.

It was possible that John would die in that institution and no one apart from the employees would know he was gone. But I would know. His friends at the group home would know. God would know.

I lifted the photo. Three boys and a girl stood erect, their parents sitting in the foreground. I turned it over and saw that the children's names and ages had been carefully penned across the back with a faded date inscribed in the corner, 1965. Fourteen-year-old John stood just to the left of his mother, his right hand resting on her shoulder. An awkward smile creased his face.

This family riveted me. According to John's file, the disease reared its ugly head not long after that photo was taken. A normal family, captured on film, until a mental-illness monster crawled beneath the bed of their youngest son. The photo, a carefree gathering of a family before the apocalypse of John's adolescence. For most youths, watershed moments signified the day braces were unbracketed, a driver's license was snagged, or their virginity was relinquished in the back seat of Dad's Oldsmobile. But not for John.

My eyes were fixed on his endearing dimples, dirty blonde hair, and Dennis-the-Menace cowlick. Squinting at the photo, I searched for any specter of disease lurking behind his placid face. Life could be so unfair. My father always cautioned me that "fair" (fare) was what one paid to board a bus. In other words, there was no such thing. That nugget of wisdom came from a man who spent his youth in poverty during the Great Depression and was reared by unspoiled men who were rugged self-starters. His mother died when he was five, still in kindergarten. *Kindergarten, for God's sake.*

But Dad, some lives are way less "fair" than others.

My father didn't think his circumstances were unfair. He didn't have time to even consider the possibility as a youngster. Eventually, he had a business to run and a family to feed. Dad's generation didn't have the luxury to make a fuss about their degree of happiness.

My heart ached for John. I didn't understand much about his type of mental illness, but symptoms typically appeared in late adolescence and could emerge from a combination of genetics, environmental factors, brain chemistry, and other illnesses. The information about schizophrenia was inadequate in the 1960s and '70s, and the ignorance and stigma prevalent back then would've made the diagnosis a brutal reckoning.

Perhaps John had been unloaded upon the group home by an angry and frustrated family who had tried every medical and social option—like the young, overwhelmed teenager who abandoned her newborn to a random doorstep under the cover of night. A good person whose long-standing patience for the snares of life had run low, as it likely did for John's family. He had now landed on my "doorstep." So I invited him in from an unforgiving and, at times, heartless world.

I removed my moist mask and sang to him. I chose a hymn that I was weary of hearing at funerals, but its theology was scriptural and instructive. It taught us that what we can *see* in the world at any given time depended on the state of our inner being. So our perspective on the affairs of the world depends on our level of spiritual maturity, our emotional IQ, and our integrity.

Unfortunately, that explains a lot.

Jesus once said, "Take the *log* out of your own eye, so you can see clearly enough to take the *speck* out of your neighbor's eye" (Luke 6:42). Our Buddhist neighbors called the log-removal process "lens-wiping." Perhaps chaplains and pastors were somewhat like ophthalmologists then: We helped our clients remove "splinters" from their eyes to bring the grainy truth into focus. I've learned that staring reality squarely in the face and surrendering to its adjustments does bring contentment, and even joy, eventually.

I halted mid-verse when John turned toward me.

"Don't be afraid. My name is Maryclaire. I'm your chaplain." John's eyes were the hue of hazelnuts with flecks of green.

"Do you feel any pain?"

He nodded. "My back hurts."

"Can you show me?" He reached for his lower back.

I paged our hospice RN. His eyes stayed locked on mine.

"I'm dying."

"Yes." I waited a beat.

"And no."

Confusion clouded his certainty. "Your body is dying, but your soul is very much alive," I explained. "In fact, your body is struggling to bring forth your soul." I've always found the birth analogy to be apt for what was really happening during the physical act of dying.

"None of that matters," he mumbled. "There are no good prospects for me. I'm going to hell."

I had assumed that he was already well-acquainted with the harrowing realities of hell on earth. After all, his life had been such an arduous, lonely, and dark journey.

"Why would you say that?" I leaned toward him.

"Lots of people figured that to be true . . . and said so . . . in those exact words."

He paused. "Well, not my mother."

"No, of course not, a good mother would never utter such a thing."

"I never had friends, really. I didn't trust people, so I mostly stayed to myself. My only real friend was my horse, BB."

We both inhaled the medicinal properties of the eucalyptus-infused room. My stomach had settled. I retrieved a bottle of water from my tote.

"BB, like in a kid's air rifle?" I inquired.

"No, BB is short for Bilbo Baggins, you know, the hobbit. He was a good guy." He gestured toward the bookshelf.

"I've read about that 'good guy' and really enjoyed the story. Do you think you're a good guy?"

"I tried to be, but those people were probably right . . . about hell. I did some awful things. I didn't mean for bad things to happen. I felt threatened, so I got defensive. My family took the brunt of it all."

During a bad storm, John explained, thunder had roused him from a restless sleep. He had heard a muffled thud, and his first instinct was to grab the cutlery knife off his dinner plate beside the bed. Lightning flashes only intermittently broke up the darkness, and he didn't recognize the figure at the top of the stairs. John lunged toward the person.

At that point, he hadn't known his older brother had rushed upstairs to warn him of severe weather approaching and had tripped on an uneven carpet tread, which caused the mysterious noise. John tried to reassure me, or maybe himself, that the knife wound had been more or less superficial. His brother got stitched up "just fine."

John turned to gaze at the crumbling ceiling tiles as if they were puzzle pieces that needed placing. Long, white greasy strands of hair burrowed behind each ear. I lowered my gaze to his hands. The fatty tissue of his right palm was shiny and ridged with thick calluses, the nail beds reddened and raw. Nicotine stained his right thumb and index finger.

"Got a smoke on ya?" His abrupt request startled me.

I imagined myself retrieving two "coffin nails" from a pack in my purse and leaning in to offer him a light. Within reason, we allowed our patients to enjoy cigarettes, alcohol, or sweets. Those vices could no longer inflict harm on lungs, livers, or heart valves. Or hasten death. Not this late in the game. Perhaps allowing him a beer on the patio wouldn't hurt but we had already started the supplemental oxygen. So, I explained to him the danger that smoking cigarettes posed for him and his roommate.

What other comforts might I substitute for John? Rumi's prediction of the revelation of "secrets at dawn" might not see the light of day unless some type of fellowship was formed between us. A chaplain carried many tools and methodologies for pastoral counselling. A smoke and a beer, along with Bible verses were appropriate resources for some patients.

John continued, "I stole stuff . . . got caught with drugs . . . beat up a neighbor kid. In my defense, though, he was a bully." Before I could respond to John's litany of offenses, he closed his eyes.

Rumi, you cautioned me at dawn about the secrets and new opportunities that would be revealed today. I was suspicious. But you were right. This was a day made to order for confessions and concessions.

Rumi was one of my favorite mystics because he stated ideas that should be evident but weren't always obvious when a person was mired in the muck of a thorny dilemma. The mystic spouted truisms like, "Don't search for water while you're standing in a stream." I could relate to wading into a surging stream up to my thighs and still searching for water. Rumi was one of the Persian poets that described how to unpack the spiritual importance of every experience, whether good or bad.

What did it mean to "unpack" a spiritual experience? Winston Churchill shed light on what it was *not*. He once said, "Man will occasionally stumble upon the truth [about himself], but most of the time, he will quickly pick himself up and keep going."

My role as a chaplain was to help people pause at the truth about themselves. As an end-of-life guide, I supported my patients through the stage of biological deconstruction and its accompanying emotional and spiritual disorder and restructuring. Everyone must do their own soul-work, but it helps to have a like-minded spiritual companion at one's side. Alan D. Wolfert, Ph.D., noted, "Companioning is about going to the wilderness of the soul with another human being, but it's not about thinking you are responsible for finding the entire way out for anyone." *Thank God.*

For a person to be a sound spiritual companion for the wounded, the wounded minister or lay person can only help if their own soul-work has been initiated. "Wounded healer" was a term created by psychologist Carl Jung in 1951. The earlier we attend to our own emotional and spiritual work, the less harm we inflict on others, and the less baggage we need to examine at the end of our lives.

Rohr said, "As we go through life—the rejections, failures, betrayals, insults, and bad choices contribute to our wounds piling up." For people like John, traumatized by a mental illness in adolescence, sorting it all out was an even harder uphill battle. Soul work on earth is crucial. I believe that our quality of life here and in the next world depends on it.

Rohr continued, "There is no nonstop flight or easy path to enlightenment [inner-harmony, wholeness, heaven]. Getting there is the insistence on going *through* reality—not *under, over,* or *around it*. If we are blessed enough to become 'stalled' in a disordered stage, there can be no cover-up, no hiding, no denial, and no addictions." Like a car that stalls because some interior part needs attention, the situation that precipitates a stall in our own lives forces us to take stock of things. Unfortunately for John, life had kept him stranded and stalled in a severe mental disease.

A Bullshit Barometer

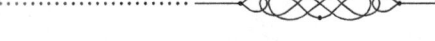

"God allows us to experience the low points in life in order to teach us lessons that we could learn in no other way."

CS Lewis, British writer and Anglican lay theologian

THE FACILITY RN ARRIVED TO TAKE JOHN'S VITAL SIGNS. I had phoned our weekend on-call nurse about his back pain. She was an hour away with another dying patient. She advised the facility nursing assistant to start the comfort kit until she arrived.

A hospice comfort kit is a small supply of medications kept on the unit or in the home to rapidly treat symptoms that occur in a patient who is dying. It contains morphine for pain and shortness of breath, atropine drops to dry secretions in the airway, and lorazepam for agitation and terminal restlessness, among other palliative care drugs. Those drugs were designed to combat suffering. I called it the cavalry kit.

The nurse left to retrieve the kit, but ten minutes later, still hadn't returned. While we waited for relief, John thankfully dozed off and I sank back in my chair. A requirement for my graduate degree in religious studies was a formal "lens-wiping ceremony." An emotional "dying-before-death ritual," or destruction of the "small and false self." Take your pick. The requirements weren't listed in the course descriptions, but the theology faculty made sure they were included in our spiritual formation during the full-time, twelve-month program.

For me, preparing for chaplaincy was an eye-opening, spiritual boot camp. My theology professor told our class that we were useless to our patients, families, or students if we didn't look at our own pretenses first. I nodded with sublime naivety. *What pretenses?* Apparently, I'd gotten too accustomed to my "small and false self." Whatever that means. With a gleam in her eye, the professor (one of my favorite nuns) delivered the Enneagram typology survey to our class one dreary day. That spiritual tool of nine distinct personality types was a system that exposed one's shadows and a tendency for acting out from one of the seven capital sins or vices—greed, sloth, lust, envy, gluttony, wrath, and arrogance or pride.

The system served pastoral counselors, church leaders, educators, and, really, everyone by helping them recognize their spiritual limitations and also the opportunities for personal growth. That explanation sounded innocuous enough, but at its core, the Enneagram was a finely tuned bullshit barometer designed back in the fourteenth century or earlier. It posed as a full-length mirror that reflected every personality defect, ego defense, character flaw, and spiritual warts for the unsuspecting admirer just wanting to check a hairstyle or hemline. And with a depth so vast it could rival the wardrobe in *The Chronicles of Narnia.* One could get lost within its spiritual diagrams and mathematical formulas for weeks.

Examining the results of the survey I took that day was a brutal experience, but I needed to face things about myself. I was in my late forties when I first encountered the Enneagram. That spiritual tool forced me to halt at "the truth of myself" that I had shrewdly learned to cartwheel over by staying busy. The Enneagram survey was not your employer's Myers-Briggs Type Indicator or the StrengthFinder assessment. Those inventories are necessary and valuable and help reveal strengths, talent, skills, psychological preferences, and personality types, but the Enneagram gauged spiritual maturity and self-awareness. Human beings could possess tremendous talent, strengths, and skills but still be emotionally immature and lack self-awareness and spiritual maturity.

A perfect metaphor for going through a CliffNotes process for conversion (a spiritual reconstruction) was the iconic story of *The Wonderful Wizard of Oz* by L. Frank Baum. As the story goes, The Wizard had hoodwinked Emerald City citizens for a generation about his identity. One day, Dorothy's dog, Toto, tugged at a flimsy curtain and exposed The Wizard, who had been struggling to hide decades of deceit from the citizens and himself.

The Wizard batted at the controls in desperation, his voice exploding through the microphone, "Pay no attention to that man behind the curtain." He tried to placate his visitors through distraction. Dorothy and her friends didn't fall for the sham. They understood exactly what was before them—a pitiful little man who was controlling, domineering, self-centered, and possessed an excessive need for admiration. The textbook definition of a narcissist.

A Franciscan nun once told me that the best spiritual direction in life is a healthy marriage. My husband and I tried to hold each other emotionally accountable. In other words, we helped one another rise above self-serving bullshit.

The Enneagram was a brusque and undiplomatic unveiling of my darkest shadows and tendency to judge others. We all cling to false images of ourselves. The personality traits and character flaws we develop throughout our lives are defensive measures for survival in a competitive and unkind world. I prayed for personal growth for years, so, on cue, the Enneagram survey arrived at my theology classroom disguised as an intriguing puzzle with a voluptuous bow. Be careful what you pray for.

As I got older, those false perceptions, feelings, and artificial masks I adopted prevented my growth. Unlike The Wizard, I realized I had veered off course in my forties and then stalled again in my fifties. I hadn't grasped how "off the mark" I had wandered in my perfectionism and pride. When I was stressed or triggered, my gifts dimmed, and my vices crept forward.

That spectrum of analysis chastened me for careers in education, chaplaincy, speaking, parish leadership, and hospice advocacy work. Basically, the Enneagram allowed me to clearly see "the warts" in myself that many others already saw in me. However, allowing my shadows to show themselves, know them, and tame them would be a lifelong holy grail.

Spirituality and Religion

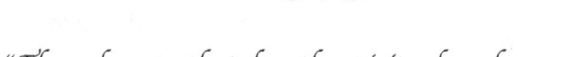

*"The only map that does the spiritual worker any good
is the one that leads to the center of the heart."*

Christina Baldwin, writer, speaker, and spiritual teacher

As I observed John, I knew his preoccupation with hell would prevent him from dying comfortably. Pain increased when a person was anxious, afraid, and tense. Research has shown that patients who work with a chaplain or pastor experience a more comfortable dying process. Many of my patients were not religious, but we all benefit from conversations about a sense of purpose, the meaning of life, our legacy, self-worth, and emotional wounds.

An aide entered, so I took the opportunity to stretch and seek the employee lounge. I called Mark with an update and relayed that I'd be home later than planned.

"No problem," he reassured me. "We decided to go fly-fishing. We just parked." Mark was on the buddy system since his solo fly-fishing expedition and subsequent heart attack on the Mississippi River. Since his triple-bypass surgery and acute damage to his heart, he had curtailed his fishing and hunting adventures. But not by choice.

My husband was not one to let a crummy day go to waste, although the rain had let up. I pictured our black Labrador, Maya, standing guard on the shore and Tom, Mark's brother, a few paces away, sitting on a stump organizing lures and rods. Mark would be hip deep in the gurgling stream, debating whether to use a dry fly or a wet fly to tease a wary trout out of a riffle. I stifled my anxiety about his daunting prognosis and reminded him about our pizza.

After placing chunks of cheddar, crackers spiked with rosemary, and an apple on a paper plate, I perched my glasses, dug out the laptop, and digested research on schizophrenia. According to an article by two eminent psychologists, people with schizophrenia had a missing "sensory-gating system," a neurological process that filters out unnecessary stimuli in the brain. As a result, auditory hallucinations, hearing voices, and other delusions may occur. The disruption of neural activity that influences brain development both prenatally and during adolescence can cause mental illness.

Schizophrenia must be one of the most challenging illnesses to cope with because it forces people to live in their heads much of the time. When a chaplain works with the soul, what does that entail? The soul is the mingling of thought, memories, insight, imagination, purpose, a sense of meaning, intelligence, feelings, and conscience. Because of that, patients with severe mental illnesses and dementia are often robbed of their claim to full humanity.

How would I help a man locked in his mind, misunderstood, and treated as insignificant most of his life restore a sense of worthiness in a few days? How would I help him understand how much God loved him?

When I re-entered the room, the disease was gaining on John's body. Death was advancing faster than we had anticipated. I untangled the damp sheets from around John's feet and saw signs of mottling. His fingertips were dusky. The purple blotches, signs of oxygen deprivation, had advanced toward his ankles, knees, and hands—a signal that blood was not reaching his extremities. The circulation system was pooling its meager resources of blood to shield John's internal organs from damage. I envisioned generals sitting at a card table, in a war room, deep in John's brain planning strategies to circumvent his death. The body is an amazing physician. It never gives up on itself. Sometimes that makes it harder to die naturally.

The LPN from the nursing home had arrived to check on John—without the emergency comfort kit in tow.

"Where's the kit, Jean?" I asked.

"It's expired." Her cheeks flushed.

"Excuse me?" I counted to twelve and reminded myself that she was only the messenger.

"What do you mean . . . 'it's expired?'" My tone remained neutral, but deep within me, my blood pressure understood the score.

"Apparently, your hospice RN neglected to check the expiration date and reorder," she announced boldly. She was not about to accept an ounce of blame for our medical failure. Good for her. Nursing homes are considered the primary caregivers of hospice patients, but this major slip-up was on us.

We'd encountered a high turnover rate of our best RNs in the last four months, and the new RN was as green as an unripe banana. But the patient shouldn't suffer because an inexperienced and uncertified hospice team member was cutting her teeth on a new job. I paged our on-call hospice nurse *again* and left a message: *Urgent. Morphine. ASAP. We have no comfort kit.* I left a message for our on-call medical director about a new prescription as well.

Plan B was that we offer the supplies we had on hand. I fetched a heated blanket and cold compresses for John's face and neck. More heavy-duty Tylenol. Paltry measures, at best. Mistakes happened, but this was not a mistake—this was negligence. The only mission for a hospice company was to prepare the terminally ill for a comfortable death. It was their only raison d'être and they get paid big bucks. I'd let our on-call RN deal with the comfort kit fiasco. I needed to focus on the spiritual and religious aspects of John's care.

Some families declined chaplain services during admission onto hospice while explaining that their loved ones were not "spiritual." I tried to explain the distinction between "spirituality" and "religion."

Secular spirituality is a vital component of what it means to be human. There are five dimensions inherent in each of us: spiritual, intellectual, emotional, social, and physical. When death approaches, most people want to explore their lives and what their legacies might entail. Chaplains, death doulas, and social workers assist with those examinations.

The spiritual dimension of the human person is about how we live with purpose and meaning; it is unique to each of us. People search for it through the arts, nature, travel, careers, social causes, hobbies, raising families, sports, meditation, religion, or a combination of these. The role of a hospice chaplain is not to convert a patient to one religion, belief, or perspective before they die. We would be fired. We take our cues from the patient.

Many people do not find meaning in this life through a particular religion—its dogma, doctrine, liturgies, sacred writings, or religious community. A 2021 Gallup Poll reported that fewer than half of US adults surveyed belonged to a church, synagogue, or mosque highlighting a dramatic trend away from religious affiliation. But 85 percent of my patients described themselves as "religious" or belonging to a religious community among one of the five major religious traditions: Hinduism, Buddhism, Judaism, Christianity, and Islam. Of those, 75 percent described themselves as Christian.

The rest identified themselves as agnostic. An agnostic believes that nothing can be known of the existence or nature of God, and therefore claims neither faith nor disbelief. We are all in different places on the spectrum of faith development and hope. I had a few families decline chaplain services for loved ones who were self-identified atheists. My role as a chaplain was not to evangelize or proselytize. I respected the Holy Spirit who works differently in each life and utilized the specific scriptures for my patients who believed in God: Jewish scriptures, Christian testament, the Quran, or, in the case of Indigenous peoples, a translation of Christian texts by

Indigenous peoples that embraces their tribes' traditions, storytelling, and language. As well, I tried to incorporate their native rituals.

The notes in John's chart indicated he was Episcopalian. When he awoke, it would be time for us to have a more in-depth conversation about his religious beliefs.

Hell is in Your Mind

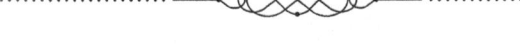

The Jesuit Order identifies hell as "an emotionally painful state, but not a sulfurous place."

"Do you want to talk about anything?" I asked, pushing my chair closer to John's bed.

"Do *you* think I'm going to hell?"

My jaw hardened. That question always made me sad coming from a good-hearted person like John.

"You know what I think? You are not 'going' to hell, despite the opinions of your neighbors. Second, hell is not a place. Rather, it is a state of existence that is the opposite of all that is whole, hopeful, joyful, and compassionate. Not an ounce of love exists in the head-heart space that is hell.

"John, I can't imagine you willing to separate yourself from the Ultimate Comforter and Benefactor. From the Truth. Although, seeing the searing truth of a thing is a hard pill to swallow for everyone. And hell is a state of such total alienation and darkness that a merciful, forgiving God would never want anyone to choose it."

"You describe it as if you've been inside my mind," John said. "Who would purposefully choose that? To suffer like I did for my entire life. Misunderstood . . . and alone." He was shivering.

"It seems unimaginable to me, too." I tucked the blanket around his shoulders.

I reminded him that he was born with an illness that disrupted the proper functioning of his brain and impaired his thinking, which in turn, affected his behavior.

"It's difficult to bear moral responsibility for choices when your brain is not functioning properly, and the victims of your malfunctioning brain didn't have it easy either." I could tell he was digesting those facts and stressing over the implications.

"It wasn't supposed to be like this," I mumbled to myself, but he heard me.

"What wasn't?"

"Damn it to hell," I uttered in frustration, thinking about the whereabouts of the comfort kit.

"Chaplains swear?" Despite his mounting pain and weakness, slight amusement sparked his eyes. I think my use of profanity helped endear me to him. Whatever works.

"Yes, chaplains swear. But usually not in front of patients."

Our policies and protocols had recently strayed from the company's original mission and, therefore, our care was slipping. So, yes, I had explained to John that when I was severely frustrated a favorite cuss word often hit the bull's eye.

A well-placed expletive was like a quick dip, a thirty-minute chair massage, or listening to a Gregorian chant. But short of that, a juicy curse muttered through clenched teeth, or even one loud enough to foul the surrounding air, reduced on-the-spot stress for a chaplain in crisis. A mini-vacation with my husband to relieve work-related stress seemed appropriate right about now. I thought about the pizza and Stella that awaited my return.

Now back to John's original question.

"Ah, yes. What was life supposed to be like?" I turned back the clock 13.8 billion years: beyond woundedness and even further back to the period of genuine innocence, or as theologian Matthew

Fox once described it, "The Original Blessing." When two plus two equaled four.

"Beautiful . . . it was supposed to be beautiful. And meaningful . . . full of purpose. It was meant to be inspirational, creative, and free. And steeped in wholeness. It was supposed to be hospitable, safe, and fair. And, of course, challenging. The Garden of Eden would never be boring. We all lived together in harmony—beasts, beauty, and humans alike. Everyone belonged. Everyone. No specter of death, dread, or suffering hovered anywhere."

I realized I was describing life beyond "the Thin Veil." But for me, the core element of how "it was supposed to be" was that we knew authentic love. And we acted like we knew it.

"But then it got all messed up. Spoiled, like curdled milk. God's gift of free will was the culprit. It seemed beyond our ability to cope. So, we threw away our kid gloves, and innocence flew out the window." John didn't respond. Was he thinking or sleeping?

Suddenly, he groaned, trying to face me. Agony deepened the wrinkles on his forehead. The prospect of grappling with existential issues with John while he was in pain and we waited for palliative medication was inciting my anger. But I had no recourse. So I continued, as I held his hand.

In some way, I believe our life on earth is a beautiful foretaste of heaven. But surmising that most of his life was lived in the twisted jungles of his mind, I assumed he was only familiar with constant danger and darkness. However, no matter what hardships this world dishes out, we should also be aware of the joy it provides.

Fortunately, chaplains had assorted tools like "spiritual machetes" at their disposal to help people make room for light and hope. In the dream world, the machete was a symbol for cutting through the underbrush of life—those gnarly thickets that kept us entangled in emotional immaturity, prevented healthy growth, and the possibility of something newly seeded to find room to blossom.

We sat in silence for a long while before John finally opened his eyes. "You should call me Johnny," he said matter-of-factly. Where did that idea come from? A grin brightened my face.

Sharing morning secrets must nurture trust. Ah, Rumi.

"Tell me what you were most grateful for in life, Johnny. What gave you joy?" Soon, comforting memories seemed to jar his lethargy and distract from discomfort, and his face relaxed a bit. It had been over an hour since I had placed my plea for assistance with our RN.

"I loved to ride. It was the only time I felt free. When I couldn't stand being in my own skin, I'd saddle up Billy and head to the edge of our property—eighty acres out—toward the ridge. Abel's Hill, we called it, named after my maternal granddad. Man, I could sit up there for hours just thinking . . . or sketching . . . with a stub of charcoal that I kept in the cigarette pocket of my vest."

Distraction had helped to calm him. Those memories emanated from his heart. *That's it, Johnny. Stay out of your head.*

"I could see everything from that ridge: acres of fields, forests, our barn and paddocks, even the old stone homestead. I'd watch the combine harvest the corn, wheat, and soybeans. The balers spit out bundles of silage across the landscape—the process was so orderly, predictable . . . and productive. Everything I wasn't. But sitting on that ridge helped to ground me. I felt more human up there, like I was rooted deep within the moist earth."

Johnny hacked up a glob of greenish phlegm and grabbed for his stomach. I retrieved my gloves and wiped his mouth and chin. His lower airway must be inflamed. We also needed the atropine drops. *This situation was not what hospice was advertised as or "supposed to be." On the other hand, was anything in life what it was "supposed to be?"*

Schizophrenia

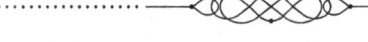

"When I was a boy and would see scary things, my mother would say, 'Look for the helpers.'"

Fred Rogers, Presbyterian minister and television host

"Y OU SKETCH." I PRODDED.

"It was my favorite class in high school. It kept me from thinking."

I nodded. I understood that, too . . . the need to take breaks from residing in my head.

"What did you sketch?" I glanced at the bookshelf, hoping for a shred of artwork on display.

"Silence. Stillness. Desolation. I sketched moods, mostly." He noticed my puzzled look. "I know that seems odd. Real artists draw the particulars of a landscape." He tried to move to gain some physical comfort, but the increasing pain enveloping his middle only produced a moan under the shifting of his weight.

I paged the facility RN to see about using a Tylenol suppository.

That comfort kit must be arriving by stagecoach. Damn it to hell. Whatever happened to timely pain management and comfort? We owe him that much. He had suffered enough.

As the afternoon stretched on, remaining present and speaking demanded more of his effort, but he evidently needed to say his piece.

"I understood winter: its darkness and death, its melancholy and loneliness. The farm was beautiful in that season. So stark. Severe. Wind-swept and naked. Winter squeezed everything to death. I felt akin to it."

He was so articulate when speaking about his feelings and art.

I told Johnny that he was a *real* artist. The real deal. Observant. Honest. Imaginative. Intuitive. Passionate. He made people feel certain things. He sketched schizophrenia as a season and created a landscape of what mental illness felt like. Johnny provided hope, just like God. He did experience what it was "supposed to be like" in a manner that many people never do.

"I'm thirsty," he whispered.

Johnny had trouble swallowing now, so I took an oral-care swab out of his water glass and moistened his gums and lips. He nodded in gratitude, like the polite cowboy who tipped his hat to a lady in the movie *True Grit*. I thought of Christ on the cross and explained to Johnny how the soldiers saturated a sponge with diluted vinegar and gall (attributed to the poppy plant), attached it to a reed, and raised it to his lips. But by refusing to drink it, a narcotic that would've numbed his pain, He chose to experience the worst of human misery. Jesus understood suffering. The demands of it, the depth of it, the isolation of it.

I pondered this hardened cowboy's penchant for sketching melancholy and winter-stricken months. "Did you ever sketch the season of spring?"

"Nah, spring is for a second stab at life. A season for optimism and lightheartedness." In low, halting tones, he described living with schizophrenia like it was a type of Groundhog Day; a never-ending feral winter.

"Do you wanna know what I always wished for?" he asked.

"Of course."

"I wished that I could start my life over . . . from scratch . . . with a healthy brain, like other people."

I reached for his arm. He closed his eyes as if to shut out the notion while I searched the sky: a swath of gray, muddled clouds. Just then, Johnny's lunch tray arrived with a mechanical soft diet: soup, mashed banana, and yogurt. He couldn't really eat but he was still on the kitchen's radar.

"Have you kept any of your drawings?" I would've given anything to see what inspired his soul as a younger man.

"My mother put them in a shoebox for safe-keeping. She told me she bound them with one of her favorite hair ribbons. The choice of silk expressed something special, huh? Something she couldn't say aloud to me."

"Yes, silk is a special fabric," I said. "Beginning in the Han Dynasty, silk was a major catalyst in bringing China out of isolation. Because China guarded secrets about silk production for many centuries, silk was perceived as a miraculous fabric." Guarded secrets and people living in isolation needed coaxing with a soft touch. With silk. Tenderness and love. Like Johnny.

"She died when I was twenty-six. I placed my sketches in the casket with her, right over her heart. It was my way of apologizing for all my wrongdoing. I had to make that clear to her. For six months after she died, I worked the fields side by side with my dad until he kicked my ass out of the house." He rubbed his unshaven face with a trembling hand.

"I deserved it. He must've considered me an unpleasant and never-ending chore. I guess he had me pegged right. I had it coming."

"Do you think he had you 'pegged right?'"

"Sure, my dad was a shrewd man. I had a reputation, and I never earned my keep in his view. So, yeah, he had me pegged just about right."

"Maybe kicking you out was really an act of love. Of wisdom. Perhaps he understood you needed more support and medical help than he could offer. Did *you* ever feel as if living at the farm was a dead-end . . . or that you were stuck? Sometimes, a guy has to move on to continue to grow."

"My father was no Gandalf." His jaw clenched.

"I don't believe anyone has a father as courageous, self-sacrificing, and wise as Gandalf. Well, we actually do . . . the Divine Creator."

He asked if I thought it was a dead-end living at the farm.

"Honestly, Johnny, I don't know. Sometimes it's hard to know if a person is stuck. I just know that at times, I was stuck—at a dead-end—but I didn't notice."

We sat quietly. I don't know for how long, each turned inward . . . preoccupied. He broke the silence. "The farm was my only home. I belonged there. Why would I leave?"

"Did you go to the group home after you left the farm?"

"Nope, I kicked around for a while. I didn't have a place of my own. I bunked in with relatives. Did some camping."

"When did you move there?"

"I'd gotten into trouble again and had no choice. Just so you know, I lived there for twenty-eight years. My only address for twenty-eight godforsaken years."

"What was it like?"

"Okay, I guess. Way better than a jail cell." He searched his nicotine-stained fingers. "Well, they were really strict on pill-taking which was a good thing." He paused.

"During that time, I completed my GED. I took a mail-order art course. I read. The guys were all right. I cooked some and tried to set the table like my mom. She would've been proud of my place settings. She was good at stuff like that, too. I even taught the guys how to sketch with charcoal; they called it our weekly art therapy. The worst of it? They had to sell BB." His eyes watered.

"Oh, Johnny. I'm so sorry. How did you ever replace his companionship?"

"I didn't. I sketched him. At least, who I remembered him to be . . . what he was to me."

"Did you sketch his physical likeness?" I wondered aloud.

"I tried to capture him on paper so I wouldn't forget what he looked like. But an artist can't draw a subject without integrating a part of its personality and nature, so a bit of both, I guess."

"How did you capture his spirit, Johnny?"

"BB was uncomplicated. He was pure, gentle, and affectionate. My protector. He behaved better than a lot of humans. I could trust him."

"What a wonderful companion God gave to you. Sometimes I get along better with animals than people too. People are wounded . . . complicated." I paused.

"Your friends at Oak Crest must miss you."

That comment registered surprise on his face, but it disappeared as a pained grimace creased his forehead. After I adjusted the nasal cannula tethered to an oxygen canister, I asked John if he'd like to rest, but he wanted to continue untangling his life despite the discomfort. So, I asked him if he had any regrets.

"I just wanted to feel normal, like other guys. You know, have a wife and a couple of kids. My own place. But then again, who wants to pass on genetic demons? It's a curse. I think my mom had it, too. But not as bad as me. We never spoke about it. But she was the only one in the house who seemed to understand me."

"Johnny, all parents pass on different degrees of psychological wounds and faulty genetics to their children. That's part of the human condition."

I offered him another saturated swab and gave him Extra-Strength Tylenol. No one will want to discuss Johnny's lapse in care at this week's team meeting.

Dark Nights

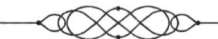

"The dark night of the soul comes just before revelation. When everything is lost, and all seems darkness, then comes the new life and all that is needed."

Joseph J. Campbell, American writer and mythologist

JOHNNY DOZED ON AND OFF IN A RESTLESS SLEEP. I HAD BRIEFLY abandoned my post to make a few phone calls, arranging a surprise that I hoped would pan out. As I reflected on my plan, he stirred and peered at me through tired, crusty eyes.

"Where *was* God?" he muttered. Johnny was still zeroed in on our previous conversation like a dog who was handed a half-chewed steak bone from the dinner table and had returned to his mat to finish the job.

I thought of that young man with the impish grin in the family photo.

"God was in your heart while you were fighting demons in your head. God was in the fertile soil on Abel's Hill. God was in the meadow and on the wings of birds flying low overhead. God was riding with you and BB as you raced across acres of barren field. God was in the moments that took your breath away. God was in your chalk-stained fingers sketching *loneliness*. God stirred a mother's heart to wrap her son's soul in silk to keep it safe. God was served at the table you so carefully set at Oak Crest. God facilitated the medical antidotes created by scientists that eased the suffering in your mind and body."

I summed it all up for Johnny. "God suffered with you. God felt exactly what you felt because God is within you. I guess the crucifixion for Jesus Christ never ends."

Johnny mustered up an insightful question. "Why not just relieve the suffering? I don't get it."

"The world can be a bitter battlefield, but God is not the cavalry. Remember, in the beginning, all was a blessing, but the precious gift of free will changed all that. God cannot undo our choices and their consequences, and God also sustains us through the victimization brought upon us by others. Real love cannot sprout and grow unless it's free. God or whatever name you prefer to call your Supreme Being (Great Spirit, Allah, Yahweh, Creator, Original Grace, Eternal Source of Life, or the Triune God) loves all of us."

For me, an apt description of how God dispensed grace was like those compact, silver parachutes that floated down to Katniss Everdeen in *The Hunger Games*. The small parachutes contained timely gifts sent during crisis—urgent necessities bestowed by a benefactor for each tribute.

Those opportune gliders dispatched to the arena, loaded with life-giving antidotes, maps, food, and survival strategies represented support, comfort, and reasons to hope during their trials in the arena. Headlamps for the darkness. However, those unmanned gliders did not have the capacity to end the tortuous games fought in the arena. I explained to John the spiritual meaning I had attributed to those parachutes.

"Did God send *me* parachutes?" Johnny wanted to know.

"Of course. Everyone gets them, and they're packed with mercy, forgiveness, and benevolence. But sometimes the resistance, friction, and the drag on them—the abuse of free will—prevents parachutes from landing on target. That is not the fault of God."

"Does God still love people if they choose to be separated from that Love?"

Johnny was a patient who kept me on my toes, but this question only required a simple answer in my mind. There was no expiration date on remorse and God's forgiveness that I knew of. Our all-loving God would never reject an ungrateful or misguided offspring like an imperfect, earthly parent might. God was patient and kind. I told Johnny that I envisioned God to be like the parent who left the porch light on to help wayward children find their way home, replacing bulbs as long as it took.

Just then, the RN, out of breath from racing up three flights of stairs, burst through the door with the medications. She explained the long delay. On the hour-long drive back to us, she got diverted to another patient who had entered the final stages of dying at another facility. And the pharmacy that we used to fill hospice prescriptions was closed. Our RN had somehow commandeered a comfort kit. None of this was her fault. We used one on-call RN on weekends to cover two huge counties, and today we had more actively-dying patients than staff.

The RN started a morphine drip and regulated the rate of flow. We usually gave morphine orally and at smaller doses, but we hadn't kept pace with Johnny's pain. Our job was to keep a tight rein on his pain, not to get into the position of trailing it. When competitors in a race get a running start, that advantage makes it difficult for the stragglers to catch up to the leaders. It's the same with pain management. And in Johnny's situation, sometimes it's challenging to get former drug abusers comfortable on the usual doses of comfort medications.

As we waited for the morphine and other drugs to kick in, I asked, "Is there anything else you need, Johnny?"

"My family," he whispered. I panicked. In his agitation, was he actually requesting their presence here?

"What about your family?" I stalled.

"Tell . . . tell them that I love them." Certainly, he didn't believe they were taking a respite down the hall littering the lounge with half-consumed cups of bitter coffee and reading outdated copies of *National Geographic.*

I promised to relay the message.

When he waved toward the tattered photograph of his family, I grabbed it and settled it into his mottled fingers. I rummaged for a piece of art from my tote portraying *Christ in the Wilderness* and stood it upright in the space once occupied by the family photo. That art piece represented where Johnny was on his spiritual path. The desert can be a place to *repent* or to turn back to something you've looked away from. Chaplain's help the dying to look back and stare down what they refused to see for most of their lives.

I explained to Johnny that he and Jesus had much in common. Jesus was misunderstood too. He bore the contempt of the Jewish religious leaders in his own synagogue, and there even came a period when his own siblings and relatives thought he was crazy. At one point, his neighbors drove him out of his village and tried to pitch him over a cliff. Jesus Christ depended on the generosity of strangers for a place to lay his head too.

I reminded Johnny that Jesus wept the night before his tortuous death—full of terror, confusion, and abandonment. And, likely, engulfed in failure. He was fully human, after all. I'm sure he had unfinished business on his mind and in his heart. We all want to finish our goals before we die.

"Stay with me," Johnny murmured.

"I won't leave you. I'll remain at your side until the only voice you hear is the one stirring in your heart."

I raised the head of his bed so he could breathe easier. Just then my cell vibrated, and I sighed in relief. Our special visitors had arrived for Johnny's final hours. It took some maneuvering, but a *parachute of grace* landed on target.

As I peered out, I saw them pacing below. I hoped it wasn't too late. I wheeled Johnny's bed to the window which jarred him to attention. When he looked down into the courtyard, he began to weep. A torrent of tears flowed from a man who had been afraid to feel for much of his life.

Just then a crew of janitors arrived with a mobile oxygen unit and escorted Johnny's bed, IV pole, and our trailing entourage to the elevator and out to the yard. Rays of light broke through the cloud cover just as a handsome stallion was led over to us. The animal snorted and whinnied.

"BB. Is it you?" Johnny commented on the white star between the stallion's eyes, the snip on his nose, and the mahogany coat. Charles, the neighboring farmer who bought BB when Johnny entered the group home, stepped forward.

"Mr. Schwartz, I want to formally introduce you to one of BB's colts, Frodo."

I couldn't help but see that the offspring was almost indistinguishable from the stallion in Johnny's photo, like Johnny and God. Johnny clung to the colt's neck. Tears of a life of mayhem mingled with the horse's mane. The small circle of misty-eyed observers smiled at the spectacle.

Passing Through the Thin Veil

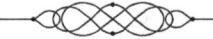

"What's lost in [physical death] is nothing compared to what's found; and all the death that ever was, set next to life, would scarcely fill a cup."
Frederick Buechner, Presbyterian minister, American author, and theologian

JOHNNY AND I WERE BACK IN HIS ROOM. ALONE. HIS BREATHING was shallow. The morphine had yet to cover all the pain. He suffered enough in this life, and he had yet to be fully relieved of it. Our one job was to keep this man comfortable. This was more than *unfair*. We bungled it. I remembered Cicely Saunders's promise. "We will do all that we can to help you die peacefully."

I didn't understand why our company no longer seemed to carry that torch. If a medical business can't maintain its mission, then it should close. Despite my heartbreak, I reminded myself that Johnny was spiritually comfortable and emotionally at peace for the first time in his complicated life. I had done my job. The palliative medications had made a moderate dent in his pain, but our lengthy delay demonstrated failure on our part. At least, he was less restless.

"What's on the other side?" Johnny murmured.

"On the other side is your true self. And I'd like to imagine that at the moment of biological death there occurs a great sense of relief; our pain is gone, and the burdens of life no longer weigh us down. Joy, justice, and light greet us. Care, comfort, and compassion filter down through our souls like salt sprinkled over popcorn. On the other side is belonging, contentment, and wholeness."

My former spiritual director introduced to me the term, "The Thin Veil." She added it as a metaphor for the doorway to heaven; a permeable sliver of chiffon between those who have passed on and those left behind. I believe that our loved ones are closer to us than we realize.

For Johnny, it will be perpetual springtime. Serenity instead of shame. I assume eternal life is more predictable and rationale than living on earth. And I've always felt certain that we will have satisfying work there, but without all of the hassles. We will pursue goals, strive, and be productive. Mostly, there will be no need for Johnny to lug around the burden of a faulty sensory-gating system.

He settled farther down into the bed. Comforted, perhaps.

"Forgive yourself, Johnny. God forgave you long ago. God evaluated the choices you made from your heart. Not the ones from your imperfect mind." You can trust God to get that right.

"Which door do I go through?"

Good question. He was pondering the portal to eternal life. I described the divine portal by borrowing a pleasant proposal of it by British author Stephen Graham. I asked Johnny to close his eyes and join me in a guided-imagery exercise.

"As you sit on the hillside, or lie prone under trees of the forest, or sprawl wet-legged by the stream at the edge of the meadow, the great door, that does not look like a door, opens."

"I'm still not sure what to look for," Johnny mumbled.

I rummaged for a New Revised Standard Version of the Bible to give him a more detailed map of what he could expect. I turned to the Gospel of John (14:27) and read, "Do not let your heart be troubled or afraid. I am going, but I will be back to take you with me, so you will be where I am."

I explained that when Jesus left the earth after His resurrection, He promised that He would return to escort us to the heavenly kingdom. "We do not navigate the journey alone. The 'Universal Christ' *is* the door—for all of humanity.

"Johnny, you can't miss it."

Blessing Johnny with holy water, I recited the prayers of commendation. In the side pocket of my tote, I carried a pyx, a small, round metal container that held Communion. It had a crimson cross etched on its gold surface.

I lifted the host close to his face and said, "The Body of Christ, the Bread of Salvation—take and become what you have received." He couldn't swallow, so I explained I would ingest this divine life for him. What I consumed would be his spiritual portion, as well. We were one body in The Spirit.

"Johnny, you no longer search, but are found. No longer blind, but now truly see. The way is within you. The door is ajar. The womb is opening wider and wider as the labor of your soul progresses. Come on, Johnny. Push. You can do it. You're so close." *It's time.*

The shadows had crept back and collected in the corners of the room. It was four o'clock in the afternoon, and Johnny was unresponsive. I clasped his hand in mine. The apnea was more frequent. I pondered the significance of breathing. To jump-start life, infants need to inhale frantic gulps of air so their tiny bodies can transition from womb to world—and at the finish line, we face the opposite. We must muster the courage to not inhale. A tall and unnatural order.

Secrets Lie in Shadows

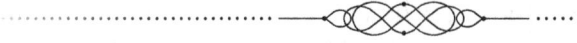

"Truth isn't found up at the top of our striving and successes, but down at the bottom in our deepest nature. By trying to climb the ladder upward, we miss Christ who comes down to us through the Incarnation."

Father Richard Rohr, OFM, American Franciscan Priest

JOHNNY HAD DIVULGED HIS SECRETS ON THAT DAY, A CONFESsion of failures and regret. But it warmed my heart to see snippets of the boy with the dimples surface in our time together. Hearing is the last sense to leave us, so I was confident he could hear me at some level. Therefore, I continued speaking to him. He was still "clinging to the bedpost" for dear life, frightened.

Families shared stories. And secrets. He and I had become like family. I think I wrote so much about Johnny because he was alone in the world, and I related to the angst of his mental illness. By far, he was the most challenging patient of my career.

So, now what do I do to help him move forward?

My own vulnerability would be my final gift to him. Professionals wouldn't share their personal stories with patients, but no one was present—only Johnny, me, and "the Escort." And the Escort already knew my story.

I told him about the severe clinical depression I suffered in my early fifties. The darkness, the emptiness, the isolation. I felt emotionally paralyzed for a year. At one point, I thought I'd never be a functioning and competent human being ever again. Challenging family circumstances, the testing of long-held values, the loss of a beloved career, family illnesses and death, and the splintering of maternal expectations (which needed some whittling) pushed me to the edge. It seemed as if the signposts that had guided me for the first half of my life were no longer applicable.

I wish I had been more resilient at that age, but my life and the religious culture were painted in black and white. Thankfully, aging has weathered most of my black-and-white certainties to the hue of gray. And soon, serious family dilemmas and health crises emerged within a span of three years. I felt as if an unraveling ball of multicolored yarn had created a web at my feet, entangling my forward motion. It was a period of my life when I feared picking up my cell phone.

Charred crimson was the hue for the hysterectomy; purple for the poignancy of an unplanned pregnancy; gray the color for disappointment when I left my beloved teaching position to go home to help my parents; indigo was the sorrow I felt watching my mother die; brown the color of bile exploding from my mouth from a dangerous bowel obstruction. Pick an ugly color; I possessed a corresponding problem.

I was barely treading water, but I guess to the outside world, I seemed to be shouldering the unrelenting responsibilities well enough. But I didn't know how to check in with myself each day, so I was unaware of my deteriorating mental and physical condition. I began to lose weight and in my frenzied state I didn't sleep much. I had unintentionally launched myself toward a steep cliff.

At first, like many of my patients, I pleaded, begged, and bartered with God to cure me. But, in time, I arrived at an understanding about my situation: I either loved God or I did not. I was either all in or I was not. I either trusted God or I did not. One day, curled up into a small despondent ball, I spoke to God with a more accommodating tone. *I changed my mind; You don't have to do anything for me.*

I love you only for yourself. I will live in any manner that gives glory to Your plan for my life. I trust you.

Between the talk-therapy, medications, rest, psychiatric visits, and emancipating my ego from my plans, I began to slowly get better. In those arduous concessions to God, I started to regain color in the complexion of my days, and a resplendent rainbow of light and hope emerged. A village of professionals came to my rescue; and that is what I wanted my hospice company to do for Johnny and all of our patients.

God had "wrestled me to the mat" for many reasons. To force me to slow down, pay attention, to look inside myself, and reflect. I was pinned. Easily outnumbered. Three to one. I lay there to ponder my options. And then I yelled, "Uncle." Afterward, God pulled me up, dusted me off, straightened my collar, kissed my cheek, and nudged me toward the door with an angel plastered to my side.

Incidentally, there can be an overlap between a clinical depression and a spiritual depression; the concept of the latter was coined "the dark night of the soul" by the Spanish mystic and poet, St. John of the Cross. Depression is a mental-health disorder, while a "dark night" is utter spiritual desolation. We all realize that life has its share of ups and downs, but when we are at our lowest, like my clinical depression, and it is coupled with a yearning for a deeper relationship with God, it is referred to as a dark night of the soul. It is considered a painful necessity for spiritual awakening.

It felt devastating to have such darkness push to the forefront of my existence. Had I lost an entire year of my life? But I came to realize what a gift God had given me. In that abysmal darkness—dank, dreary, and suffocating—I earned my most authentic credentials for chaplaincy: humility, empathy, gratitude, and a merciful spirit. Eventually, I was healthy enough to crawl up rung by rung, hand over hand—a bit worse for the wear, but on the mend. After all, I was accustomed to searching for truth in dark, dirty, and frightening places.

However, Johnny's illness had swallowed thirty years of his life. It wasn't fair, and I told him so. As I shared the painful details of my ordeal, I envisioned Johnny whispering words of encouragement as he listened to my confession and nodding in empathy as he reached for my hand. God had his back and mine. And now we had shared our secrets. And our souls.

Five minutes after I had finished telling him my story, John Adams Schwartz inhaled for the last time. I released his hand. I'd like to think that a bond kindled from sharing the burden of a mental illness had helped him to let go.

Imagine. Everything he ever wished for . . . he now possessed. No more crossroads, thresholds, and obstacles. It was clear sailing through the door that never looked like a door until he was ready to walk through it. He finished his spiritual work on earth.

I placed a fresh sheet over his body and alerted the funeral home and his legal guardian. My paperwork for the spiritual assessment was next. The Centers of Medicare and Medicaid required this documentation, as well. Our RN rejoined me in the room, and we stayed until they wheeled his body out the front door. He entered with no family, but he would leave with me, members of the hospice team, and facility staffers at his side. And, of course, accompanied by his loyal "Escort," the One who would accompany Johnny to His own residence.

I called Mark. He suggested the movie, but it no longer fit my mood. I countered with a beer out at the firepit and reiterated that I'd still take the pizza. That night, I needed to be outdoors inhaling fresh air in the arms of my husband.

While we nestled on the glider, Mark asked if I was warm enough. No one could shiver beneath a blanket of stars spun into the billions across the sky. No one who had a mother trilling exotic bird melodies from the other side of that sparkling canopy could ever feel the chill of loneliness.

Then, Mark exhaled one of those long, deep sighs of contentment and said, "When it's my turn to leave this grand universe, look for me in nature."

The next day, I visited the group home and distributed Johnny's few belongings. Three items. Perhaps they had to draw lots. I gave the funeral director the family photo and the framed picture of BB with explicit instructions to place them over his heart.

When I had gathered Johnny's belongings, two pieces of heavy-stock paper dropped to the floor from his *Hobbit* book. My hands trembled when I saw what they were. Johnny must've forgotten that he had slipped two of his smaller sketches into its pages. One depicted deer at the forest's edge, and the other, lilacs in various stages of bloom.

But these depictions of nature didn't coincide with what Johnny liked to draw, and he denied sketching landscapes or still life. I turned over the drawings, and the name of the artist was scrawled in the corner: Jane M. Schwartz. His mother had sketched. She must have placed her art there before she died. He never mentioned it. Did he know the two pieces were there? The miracle of silk and love. An enigmatic and artistic exchange between like-minded spiritual travelers. Mother and son worked out the travails of life by sketching, perhaps unbeknownst to the other.

I kept one drawing, her sketch of springtime, and put it in my Bible. Johnny would have approved. I framed Jane's rendering of the deer for the dining room wall at the group home. Only one final errand remained. Two weeks later, I drove out to Abel's Hill. Johnny had spent hours there sketching, sorting through the travails of life from his post on the ridge, just watching clusters of clouds float by. There was no designated administrator for Johnny's cremains, so after searching for the right spot, I tossed some of his ashes to the wind as a blessing upon his farm, fields, homestead, and wildlife. The rest, I buried next to his mother.

Near the end, Gandalf reported to Pippin in *The Return of the King*: "*End?* No. The journey doesn't *end here.* Death is just another path . . . one that we all must take. The gray, rainy curtain of this world rolls back and all turns to silver glass. And then you see it . . .

the white shores . . . and beyond. A far green country under a swift sunrise."

So you see, that is the role of a hospice provider—to deliver dying patients in comfort to those "white shores and that green country under a sunrise."

A Day Away from Death

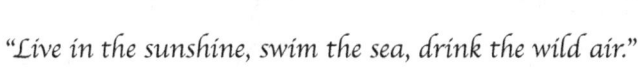

"Live in the sunshine, swim the sea, drink the wild air."

Ralph Waldo Emerson, essayist and poet

I woke to the panting of our seven-year-old black Labrador, Maya, six inches from my face. The weekend had come around again. Finally. And it was too early to get out of bed. Rebelling, I rolled over and reveled in my down comforter. Maya paced at my side, so I planted my feet onto the chilly hardwood floor and wiggled into my oversized mules. I pulled up the shade to reveal a cloudless sky.

I heard my husband puttering in the kitchen—the aroma of sizzling bacon and freshly perked coffee wafted through the house. After feeding the cats who had been anxiously circling my ankles, I went to retrieve the morning paper. I enjoyed the crimson hue of the sumac carpeting the ridge behind our home and the smoky scent of burning leaves on an autumn morning.

As I stepped back into the house, Mark's sonorous baritone soared above the steam of the shower. I filled a pan with water to poach eggs, popped in the toast, and cut sections of grapefruit while listening to the symphonic strains of Handel's *Water Music Suite* from my playlist. Perfect inspiration for a day on the lake.

Mark came into the kitchen dressed in a quick-dry, long-sleeved shirt, fishing vest, and the gray canvas pants I bought him for his birthday. We were both eager to spend a day together on the chain of lakes twenty miles west of our home. Kayaking, fishing, bird-watching, and a picnic were on the agenda. I felt just like a kid sprung from nine months of school.

Mark planted a kiss on the top of my head and grabbed the sports section. He had set the table with the blue-and-white floral dishes we had purchased when we got married. It was a deal where a customer could earn points toward eight place settings by buying groceries. Two weeks of groceries earned me a silver-rimmed gravy bowl. I was so excited to place that bowl next to my first Thanksgiving turkey. The astute businessperson who thought to marry the drudgery of weekly grocery shopping with free kitchenware was a marketing genius.

In the 1970s, most young homemakers in our town had the same generic blue and white pattern, but no one seemed to care. Our dishes served as a metaphor for our thirty-year-old marriage. Worn, a bit chipped in spots, and the sheen had faded, but dearly familiar and treasured.

"You're using our fancy dinnerware this morning," I teased. "What's the occasion?"

"You're the occasion. You're not on-call for once." He lowered the paper to show me the infamous crinkle of his almond-shaped eyes. Eyes the hue of melted caramels that I fell in love with in fifth grade.

We met at St. Francis grade school. Mark sat behind me; that was a mistake. All I can say about that first day of school and its seating arrangement is that I'm glad inkwells set into desktops were obsolete. My long blonde ponytail would've been a constant lure for a dousing in the jar of jet-black liquid. Let's just say that Mark's middle name was "Mischievous." Fortunately for me, my father had moved us from Wausau to Green Bay for his promotion in the insurance industry. That decision changed the trajectory of my life forever.

I was intrigued even then by this rugged boy with shaggy bangs that just skimmed his prominent brows. By eighth grade, I was wearing his friendship ring threaded through a tarnished chain. We were both athletic and enjoyed playing tennis, racing down ski slopes, and trekking along cross-country ski trails. Hand in hand, we walked to the local drug store on the corner of Main and Broadway, a mere block from our school. In those days the store still hired soda jerks and served up old-fashioned concoctions of syrupy cocktails called "green rivers" and "cherry phosphates."

Mark and I attended high schools in different cities, but we met up for homecoming, senior prom, sporting events, and musical productions. We were both shy in new situations, but our relationship was one of comfort, similar interests, and a solid friendship. After five years of living on opposite sides of the country in search of finding ourselves and preparing for careers, we gravitated back to our roots and each other.

Mark proposed when we were twenty-three with a one-carat diamond retrieved from a 1967 Green Bay Packers Super Bowl ring. His father, John Sr., was on the Packers' Board of Directors. When the youngest of six, Mark, was ready to fly the coop, his three older brothers had already culled diamonds from precious family heirlooms for their engagements and left the brooches barren with gaping holes. Mark's dad offered us the solitary diamond from his own dazzling ring. My engagement ring was a windfall for an avid Packer fan and diamond enthusiast like me.

Now Mark and I sat together, savoring the steaming caffeine, lost in the news of the day. I perused the entertainment page with its word puzzles and a Sudoku. After the last morsels of the meal disappeared, Mark hustled me along: "What do you say we get a move on?"

"Just give me a minute, I'm almost finished with this crossword. What is the word for '*love,*' in Latin?" He didn't answer immediately, so I glanced up.

His thick cut of an eyebrow arched to the edge of his hairline. He then raised each brow quickly in alternating succession, like Morse code. For the finale, he threw in his irresistible, impish grin. I was well-acquainted with Mark's clever telecommunications.

"Stop," I protested. He was such a clever tactician in regard to romantic proposals.

He had the most flexible eyebrow contortions that I'd ever seen and worked this talent to great advantage—usually. *Flirt*.

"No, we are not going back to bed—we are going to the beach." *Men*. Now that I was up, I needed to get *out* of the house. I feigned disdain with a smirk on my face, but laughter in my heart. I penciled the letters for "amare" in the five boxes for twenty-six across. He stood as if to say, "Okay, let's do it."

I watched him take a handful of pills, his early morning prescriptions, and shove the container of remaining capsules deep into his knapsack. Feeling blessed to have dodged death that day on the stream near La Crosse, I looked forward to a day on the water with him. Every day was a gift.

It was chilly to start—barely fifty degrees at dawn. The temperature would be brisk if we swam, so I threw our wetsuits into the tote. Mark secured the sea kayaks to the saddles on the car carrier. On the short drive down the highway, I thought about Mark's impish sense of humor.

The previous week at church, minutes before I approached the lectern to speak about the topic of stewardship, Mark whispered a quick joke. I broke out into a muffled fit of giggles, but he maintained an air of stoic composure to the slight heaving of my shoulders. My nose dripping, I laughed even harder. I could only imagine what the parishioners behind us were thinking. I was too embarrassed to look. Mark covertly passed his handkerchief while soberly singing a stanza from the Communion hymn, allegedly focused on the ritual at the altar. Yeah, right.

"Really, Mark, we're in church, for God's sake," I'd hissed. I glanced up at the statue of Jesus and pleaded in quiet desperation,

"This was the soul mate you paired me with before time began. You bear some responsibility for this."

Did I see the statue wink?

I worried about my husband. Despite Mark's weekly rehabilitation, his chest discomfort occasionally reoccurred. The cardiac experts at Mayo Clinic in Rochester, Minnesota, gave us a grim prognosis after the heart attack. Mark had "two to five years to live without a heart transplant." Watching him struggle to comprehend that prognosis and the initial despair that accompanied the four-hour drive back to Milwaukee with our daughter, Annie, was heart-wrenching. I tried to be strong and positive for him, but I was often a dismal failure.

Even though they placed Mark near the top of the Midwest transplant list, something always got in the way. A serious infection was the usual culprit. So, I awoke many mornings already stressed before the day had even begun. If I turned off the pulsating air from his CPAP machine, would he still be breathing? Once, I did unplug the machine before I left for work and I woke him up.

"What are you doing?"

"I just wanted to see if you were still alive."

This is how we lived. His father died at age seventy-three of end-stage heart disease. Mark was only fifty-seven.

The previous weekend, his defibrillator had gone off while we were spring-cleaning the garage, and the rescue squad rushed him to the nearest hospital. I had gotten accustomed to tailing the EMTs. He had disability insurance and worked part time in a job he enjoyed. I was grateful for that. On this day, I just wanted to enjoy Mark, the water, and the birds, and forget about anyone's terminal prognosis.

A boisterous refrain spilled from the car windows all the way to the boat launch, something about, "When the smelt are running on the old bay shore, I'll be singing this song to you." Mark had introduced me to fishing for smelt during the spring spawning runs on the shores of Lake Michigan in the 1980s near our newlywed cabin.

On quiet nights we sat together on the banks of the lake wrapped in wool blankets and listened for their arrival with a soft, swooshing sound. When his mother first saw our tiny abode, she muttered in disgust: "You can't bring your bride home to that. It doesn't even have central heating."

But for us, it possessed major selling points: We could keep a dog there; it sat on a gurgling stream in a dense thicket of trees; one wall was draped with a quaint, stone fireplace that always deposited its smoky malfunction to the four rooms (but romantic enough, for us); and it possessed a nifty screened-in porch that hung haphazardly off to one side. Mark was the only heat source I needed. We loved that place.

We fished for smelt at night when the water temperatures climbed to the low 40s. We used long-handled A-frame dip nets based on a Native American design. We hauled up hundreds of smelt and deep fried them in a light batter right on the banks of the Menominee River. They were five to eight inches in length and tasted of sweet cucumber and chicken. We devoured them whole—head, bones, and all. Crunchy. When Mark started in on the refrain about smelting, I knew it was time to gather our friends and head to the muddy banks of the river.

Mark and I were now driving to a special region of Wisconsin: The bodies of water are described by the locals as "lake country." The lakes were named by the most populous tribe in southeastern Wisconsin since the early 1800s, the Potawatomi. They were an Algonquian-speaking Native American people who lived in this area for four centuries. The lakes we were exploring that day were named Nemahbin, derived from the Native American word for our common fish, known as a "sucker"; and Nashotah, which means "twin." The surrounding lakes were Nagawicka, which signifies "sandy"; Okauchee, translating to "small"; Oconomowoc, meaning "gathering of the waters"; and Pewaukee, meaning "Lake of Shells."

We pulled into the parking lot and untied the straps on my kayak. I loaded the food, my phone, binoculars, and sunscreen into the dry bag. The towels, picnic supplies, my book, and a stadium blanket went into the hatch. I swapped sandals for water shoes, grabbed my visor and sunglasses, and buckled my life jacket before pushing out. As the water level deepened, I lowered the rudder.

Mark had his kayak down and was positioning his fishing equipment. I waited for him just offshore. We put in on Lower Nemahbin Lake and would navigate under a bridge to its upper portion, then paddle our way through a narrow inlet to Lower Nashotah Lake. We'd portage over a narrow bridge to reach Upper Nashotah Lake, our destination. This chain of four lakes ran straight north, in close succession, each with its unique channels, shoreline, and ecology.

Finally, Mark pushed off from the dock.

"I love you," I shouted to him.

"Love you, too," he yelled back across his bow.

Lower Nemahbin Lake is only two hundred thirty-nine acres and thirty-six feet deep, which is why it is mostly sixty percent marsh and muck. A small island sits in the middle. It's great for fishing and kayaking, but we wanted to head north toward the Interstate 94 underpass to explore its northern neighbor, Upper Nemahbin Lake. Lower Nemahbin Lake was the least bedazzling of the chain of lakes.

Motorboats crisscrossed the middle of the upper lake as water enthusiasts began to arrive for the day. Mark and I hugged the shoreline along the route north to bypass the waves that disrupted our progress. We paddled by opulent lake homes on the shores of the next two lakes that had replaced the tear-downs of the modest homesteads built in the 1970s and earlier.

We glided through stretches of lily pads and woodlands. I envisioned Potawatomi families out in their fields harvesting corn, squash, and tobacco; tapping maple trees; and gathering wild rice and berries. In the 1700s, bark-covered houses would've dotted the landscape with hazy swirls of smoke billowing upward like the offerings of incense from our Sunday liturgies cleansing the people, the surrounding land, its structures, and sacred ceremonial items.

When we first moved to the lake country area, I researched the history of the Indigenous peoples who inhabited the land. Their value system was guided by a philosophy that created balance and well-being between the people, plants, and wildlife that inhabited their surroundings. What caught my attention was that the Potawatomi were known as "the keepers of the sacred fire."

For Native Americans, living with fire was a way of life, and they understood how to work with the explosive element. Small intentional burns were an important part of Indigenous spirituality, a form of medicine to keep the land and people healthy. For them, fire acted as a spiritual messenger from the Creator. Maybe that's why folks love sitting around their outdoor firepits and indoor fireplaces; they inherently understand its primordial significance and sacredness. Its hypnotic power.

It was fascinating to discover that the Potawatomi in this area naturally managed fires until the Weeks Act of 1911. That federal act outlawed Native American fire management even though there were few wildfires when they lived freely on the land. I think the western states could learn so much from the fire stewardship of Native Americans. The Potawatomi were stewards of the land long before Wisconsin became a state in 1848.

My husband, children, and I tapped trees every year too, but we were lucky if we collected enough sap every spring to fill four one-quart bottles with syrup after boiling down gallons of sap. But our labor-intensive, annual family project for a month's worth of the natural sweetener to douse our pancakes, waffles, and French toast is a memory I still relish.

Finally, Mark and I reached the narrow sandy beach on Lower Nashotah Lake, and my musing ended. We spread out the blanket and dug out the wine, plates, fruit, cheese, salami, and a loaf of French bread. Stretched out, we enjoyed the smorgasbord and extended our faces to the early October sun—like the sunflowers of summer. We talked about our kids and grandchildren, kissed, and laughed about our escapades as younger versions of ourselves. But for the most part, this was a day to discuss the proper bait for largemouth bass and bluegills, Wisconsin bird habitats, and lakeside wildflowers. When was the last time I possessed the heart of a teenager?

Mark embarked for the lake's center, which was forty-seven feet deep, while I packed the leftovers. Spying a cove tucked under a grove of aspen just up ahead, I decided it would be a lovely place to tie up and read while Mark tried to snare the surf portion for dinner. The turf entrée, hunted last fall, thawed in the fridge. Pheasant was my favorite wild meat; it tasted of untamed wetlands, harvested grain, nuts, and sweet berries. My first meal with Mark's family was a wild-duck dinner that his family of hunters (including women) brought back from their annual trek to Saskatchewan, Canada. Mark's mother was a gourmet cook and prepared the meat with enough of the wildness left intact that I was certain it wasn't purchased from the local meat market.

I pulled up to the sandy bank, managed to clamber out without falling into the three feet of water, and attached the line to the nearest sturdy branch. Using my life jacket as a pillow, I positioned myself so I could stretch out the length of my boat. Kayaking was tailor-made for a chaplain needing a day away to relax. I sampled the pinot grigio from the leather Bota bag, a Spanish wineskin that Mark bought while traveling through Europe in college, and then settled down into the boat and my book.

I split my attention between the cruelties and novelties of eighteenth-century France and surveying the movement of my surroundings. A flash of red caught my attention, and then the song of a male cardinal floated through the trees. A hawk swooped and soared and dove for unsuspecting fish. When I looked upward, the sun dappled through the canopy of golden aspen leaves, which trembled in the wind. Beautiful black fissures scarred the ivory bark, just like the deep pleats marking the face of an eighty-year-old woman.

As I listened closely, it sounded like the leaves were whispering to one another. Aspis, the aspen tree's Greek name, meant "shield." How blessed was I to spend an hour tethered to a slender stalk of aspen while resting under its leafy protection? A "shield tree." Huh. Where would I buy such a tree? A bulwark of sturdy leaves to plant near our home to hover and protect both of us. In the end, nature won the full attention of my heart. So I stored my book in the dry bag. Waves gently rocked my boat as I contemplated my surroundings, soon lulling me to sleep.

The Card

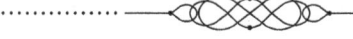

"Change will not come if we wait for some other time. We are the ones we've been waiting for. We are the change that we seek."

President Barack Obama, former US President

WHEN I AWOKE, MY ONE-TRACK MIND WENT DIRECTLY TO my last moments with Johnny, but I shook the image. As I tried to sit up, I noticed a card designed with cupids and red hearts lying at the bottom of the boat. I must've tucked it into the back of my book and forgotten about it. I reached for a Valentine's Day card dated 2005. Mark's illegible scrawl always amused me.

I kept my most-treasured cards as page markers so I could remember personal sentiments and cherished family members, and reflect on my blessings. Mark stored the letters and cards in a cardboard file labeled "Love." One day, I stumbled upon it amidst the rest of our important papers while searching for a car title in a basement filing cabinet. His romantic gesture captivated me. I'd forgotten about it until now.

> Maryclaire,
> I can date the beginning of my life to you. Before you, I cast about in search. Then came you! My safe harbor in a tumultuous sea.

> *My job is fulfilling. My family is comforting. My home is beautiful. But these are only stars orbiting around my universe—you.*
>
> *My feelings for you at the midpoint of my life have doubled those of my youth. I look forward to falling in love with you more and doubling my feelings again.*
>
> *At the end of my life, I want your hand in mine, and then I will join the stars and orbit around you forever.*

My eyes glistened while I searched for him out on the lake. As I lay back in the boat, water lapping against the port side, I considered our lives and love. A safe harbor, he had said. I watched him then—casting about—just like he mentioned in his love letter. He'd be heading back for me soon, holding up a stringer of bass with a boyish grin. I will never forget that hearty impression of him. Never. Mark sported a salt-and-pepper beard, a weathered face, and a balding scalp. As handsome as ever. My love.

I stored my belongings and untied the line. After he paddled back to me, we pulled our boats side by side so we could talk, and I offered him wine. He plucked a lily out of the water, like the corsage he proudly presented me for prom. Mark chattered about the bait and casting techniques he used to secure our dinner. Such a refreshing change—to ponder only fish for a day. I was happy to inspect his slimy trophies.

All I could think about as he shared the details of his hour-long adventure lobbing lines laden with worms was that I married a man who was more than an avid angler and bird hunter. He was a gatherer of morels and friends alike, a lover of nature, an editor, a journalist, and a visionary. But most important, he was the guy who'd go out of his way to help a person in need.

He called from his office one day to ask if a recent college graduate, a young woman he had mentored, could live with us for a few months. I gulped. Since I had just finished an academic year teaching two hundred and fifty adolescents how to negotiate the slings and arrows of high school with integrity, I needed the ten weeks of summer vacation to recharge and prepare for the next term.

I pictured Mark forming a foothold with his hands to assist this young woman's climb over the obstacles that had been strewn in her path. Obstacles mounted brick by brick by the circumstances of life, weighing her down—a mother who died prematurely after birthing a large family and a father paying a debt to society during her formative years. And finally, an adolescence frazzled by foster care.

Often, I needed to mull the personal cost and time of obstacle-clearing. Mark never did. I remember the first day the twenty-two-year-old walked into our kitchen and stoically announced, "Sometimes I have issues with white people and Catholics." I chuckled. She was two for two in describing our ethnicity and religious affiliation. I couldn't help but smile at her line of demarcation. "Me, too," I countered.

Acquiescing in the end, I taught our guest how to drive that summer. We educated one another, but she taught us and our children a lot more than we taught her. She was our mentor, not the opposite.

But my favorite of Mark's traits? For all of his pranks and mischievous spirit, he savored sincere and significant discussions about our country and the world. Mark understood the complex issues of our communities, so he started the first college-readiness program for underserved youth in the neglected neighborhoods of Milwaukee. I loved that about him.

And it was true that I provided an anchor and "safe harbor" for him. And he for me. Like kayaks on placid waters, we sailed smoothly for years in our marriage. But during a few rough patches, our marriage was put through a series of demanding challenges that churned and heaved like an angry lake—tossing us, weathering us, and shaking us—and testing our resolve. But in the end, we came 'round right. We always did.

We finally reached the end of the lake and found the channel that led into Upper Nashotah Lake. I retrieved the small marine trailer in the bow and attached it to the stern, grabbed the bungee cord at the front of my boat, and started rolling it through the thick fauna toward the next lake. I managed it myself, while Mark pulled his bulkier boat through thick underbrush by sheer muscle. Watching him, I realized he needed the handy marine trolley for portaging more than I did. Always the gentleman, he declined the offer of my trolley.

At that moment, a grimace crossed his face. *Oh, oh, this is not good*. I dropped my boat and ran back to him. Mark sank down upon the bow to catch his breath. "I'll be fine if you can just take one end."

"Should we finish here?" He had me trembling.

He brushed the discomfort aside and assured me that if we could redistribute gear from his boat to mine, the "medical annoyance" would dissipate. "Let's finish our adventure. I'll be okay," he said, dismissing the short-lived episode.

"You'll be okay, or you *are* okay?" I pressed.

He hated my wifely vigilance. I didn't care. I must've been in total denial to give in with such little protest. My go-to method for ignoring reality when I was really afraid was to continue with business as usual. We both knew we were dealing with a hot mess with his heart condition, an all-encompassing disease that would diminish the viability of Mark's other organs as it slowly eroded his longevity. But he insisted on living as normally as possible.

He seemed okay for the moment, so we lumbered on. Soon both kayaks were gliding onto the upper lake . . . the last leg of our journey. I released ten cleansing breaths.

The lake shimmering before me was my favorite of the four. No motorized boats were allowed, so we stroked smoothly and efficiently on its glassy surface, quickly covering its small area. The best non-ecological feature was that the Nashotah House Theological Seminary was built on its shore. The orthodox Anglo-Catholic campus, founded in the town of Nashotah in 1842, was a hidden treasure.

Its library and rare theological collection helped me draft my thesis toward a graduate degree in religious studies. I had enjoyed studying on the picturesque campus with its quaint, stone buildings swathed in viscous vines of English Ivy. The grounds were stunning from the water. I pointed out the chapel, library, and my favorite outdoor study areas for Mark.

This Christian denomination which allowed for the ordination of women and married priests, attracted me. In 1994, the Episcopal Church amended the church's canons to prohibit discrimination based on sexual orientation, providing equal access to the rites and worship of its church, including ordination. Catholics kiddingly referred to the Episcopalian Church as "Catholic Light." Like Pepsi Light. I had always thought that Roman Catholics should consume more of what the Episcopalians were drinking. It's nothing to joke about. If I had been born into an Episcopalian family, I might've considered ordination.

As the wind picked up, I suggested that Mark relax on the banks of the seminary grounds while I paddled back to the parking lot and retrieved our car. He shrugged.

"Or fish," I suggested. He chose the second option.

I always kept my kayak sail in the hull, so our plan called for a quick rigging of the mast to my cockpit. This would shorten my trip by half. With the wind at my back, the sail would act like a spinnaker, and I should fly to the landing. I could be back at the dock in forty-five minutes.

Mark didn't argue, his reticence speaking volumes. We both had phones, so I waved him off and navigated south. I assumed he'd be okay alone, but if he did have problems, he had a host of seminarians a stone's throw from the boat with spiritual lifelines strung straight to heaven.

I didn't plan to write about Mark in this book about hospice. He was simply an innocent bystander, the husband of an employee of HA going about the business of daily life and trying to defy his terminal prognosis. But then the reach of greed extended into our home and entangled our plans for his survival. It was then that our personal story also became fodder for another chapter.

It was grueling to live under clouds the color of gray cement and dense with the specter of death. I preferred the stalking of a luminous canopy of golden aspen leaves. Even when I didn't feel God's presence during certain periods of my life, I knew that God shielded me like that vast canopy of aspen. Sustained me. Every time, God's grace manifested through my suffering and challenging times. Come to think of it, I always matured spiritually more during challenging times than from periods of sustained comfort and stability.

Still, I envisioned the worst possible things happening to Mark to steel myself against what might transpire in those months ahead. On my way back to the dock, I envisioned Mark lying face down in the water . . . bloated and the hue of indigo. My mind was preparing me for something difficult. I could feel it in my gut.

As I drove up the road that bordered the side of the lake where Mark would be fishing, a stab of fear lingered, but he was fine. Mark sat upright in his kayak, his pole poised over lily pads and reeds near the shoreline. He grinned and waved. Smiling, I didn't know how long I could continue my constant masquerade of wellbeing.

We no longer had the energy to fillet fish, grill pheasant, and mix a salad after this unexpected extension to our day. The meal would keep. So, the day ended with a visit to a hamburger and ice cream joint called the Kiltie, a popular drive-in for families in lake country.

I remembered our dates in high school at the local A&W fast-food drive-in and sitting in the front seat of Mark's beat-up, blue Toyota, laughing hysterically at the unruly adolescent antics he shared about his all-male classrooms. Both high school and college. Material for comic storytelling was abundant with men.

We'd be okay. We had to be. He was all I knew.

Martha

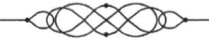

"In our attempt to banish discomfort from the world, we banish the knowledge that can save us . . . we have to learn from our illnesses, pain, secrets, and sacred spaces."

Kat Duf, writer, author, therapist.

ALL MEDICAL CHARTS BEGAN WITH A "FACE PAGE." I FLIPPED through the binder to a photo of my newly admitted hospice patient. The stoic woman stared out beyond the page, her chiseled jaw set in subtle defiance and her brow furrowed as if she goaded the viewer to dare mess with her. She had thin, white strands of hair pulled snugly to the nape of her neck. Wire rims barely contained the bulging glass framing her milky-blue eyes. Her dusky complexion, speckled with three prominent moles, sprouted black, wiry tufts of hair at her chin. She portrayed the "been around the block one too many times" type of toughness. It could pass for a mug shot.

The woman's name was inscribed in bold, black caps beneath her admission photograph, as if the size of the lettering and vividness of the type could give further tribute to her intrepid reputation. **MARTHA ELIZABETH MCCURDY,** age eighty. White female. Widow. I glanced at the medical and social work notes left by my colleagues earlier in the day. Martha was predeceased by her husband

and a daughter, but survived by a granddaughter, Katherine Louise Browne. I punched her phone number into my cell. The granddaughter answered after a few rings.

"Katherine, I'm Maryclaire Torinus . . . the hospice chaplain. Would it be all right for me to visit your grandmother today?"

She launched without preamble. "No offense, but I don't think she will get much out of your visit. In fact, if you tell her what you do up front, she may not let you through the door. Maddie and God are not exactly on the best of terms. Oh . . . and please call me Kat. Just like it sounds. K-A-T."

"Nice to meet you, Kat. But I'm puzzled. Maddie?"

"That's what they called Martha at the precinct. She was a police officer. The nickname stuck."

"How long was she an officer?"

"Thirty-five years. She was on desk duty when she retired, but before that, she was promoted to sergeant. She gained quite a reputation. You'll see."

That comment got my attention.

"Did she practice a religious tradition?"

"Yeah, somewhat. On and off, I guess. Look, it's complicated. According to my mother, when Maddie left home at seventeen, she was pregnant. Her boyfriend was back home on leave from the war, and when he went back to France, they lost touch. She grew up in an ultra-conservative, hard-core, fundamentalist home. Poor Bacia." Kat must have anticipated my confusion.

"My grandmother is mostly Polish, but she has some Native American genes, as well. I gave her a DNA kit for her birthday a while back. She's so proud of her Indigenous heritage. Anyway. My mother said they went to church together when she was a young girl. St. Rita's. A Catholic church over on Benson and Clarke. But I've never seen my grandmother even pick up a rosary. Losing my mom broke her heart. They were close. My mother was her only child."

"When did your mother die, Kat?"

"When I was seventeen . . . eighteen years ago, of cancer."

A tough age for a girl to lose a mother. "Were you close to your father and grandmother?"

"Yes, very much so. I'm doing well, married to my college sweetheart. I have a career that I mostly enjoy, working in the advertising department of a local newspaper."

Even through our cell connection, I sensed a smile forming. "The light of our life right now is our three-year-old, Liza. We call her Ladybug."

"I bet Martha loved having a great-granddaughter. I'll look for Ladybug's photos when I visit your grandmother. How often do you see her?"

"I manage to get there once a week or so."

"How does she seem to you?"

"Well, it's difficult to get a smile out of her these days. She's tired, of course, so our visits are shorter. My daughter doesn't even provoke much of a reaction anymore."

"You inferred that your grandmother and God had a 'falling out' of sorts. What happened?"

"I'd rather have her explain."

"Will she?"

I pictured Kat arching her shoulders as she responded, "I don't know, but if not, then I guess we won't need a chaplain." The dismissive comment settled on me like a not-so-subtle ultimatum. Challenges motivated me.

"Is there a specific reason you requested a chaplain when you signed the paperwork for hospice services?"

There was silence at the other end of the line. And then a robust sigh.

"She's so melancholic. And it's not just because she's dying," Kat answered. "There's more to it than that, I think. She just seems preoccupied . . . distant. It's hard to explain. I checked the box for the chaplain because I didn't know what else to do. She reminds me of those tigers pacing the perimeter of their cages—back and forth, round and round. So restless. Watching. Waiting."

"Kat, is there anything she might be waiting for?"

"I wouldn't know. Isn't that your job . . . to figure that out?"

I wondered if Kat wasn't a chip off the old maternal block. It made sense that the "acorn" wouldn't fall too far from the formidable matriarchal oak. I'd soon find out.

"I'll give it my best shot. Thanks for your help. I'll be in touch."

I informed the nurse's station that I would be visiting Martha, shoved my credentials into my jacket pocket, set my phone on vibrate, and headed down a corridor littered with peeling wallpaper and shriveled-paint chips glittering at the baseboards. The forlorn carpeting and drab walls made everyone seem feebler in this place. And somehow, even more vulnerable.

The stench of industrial-strength cleaning supplies, urine, and the remnants of lunch mingled in the air. I had yet to adjust to the distinct odor of illness and infirmity. Enthusiastic yells of "Higher!" spilled into the hallway from the iconic TV game show, *The Price Is Right*, a staple of every American nursing home. I glanced into the activity room. Boredom and fatigue sat sentry in rows of wheelchairs. Heads hung, chins to chests, drool pooling on clothing protectors.

My mortality loomed before me day after day after day in this ministry. How they looked, I would look. What they couldn't remember, I wouldn't remember. How they felt, I would feel. I stared into the stark reality of the winter of life. So, I learned to enjoy each day and appreciate every speck of health I possessed, such as the ability to thread each leg into a pair of pants without holding onto a dresser.

I replayed the comments of Martha's granddaughter in my head as I maneuvered past staff members and patients in walkers and wheelchairs. Could I make matters worse for Martha's suspicions on matters of faith? A gruff voice deep from within whispered, "Yes, you actually could." I pushed the cautionary appraisal aside.

Defiance

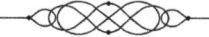

"But God is only a white cold eye, a quarter-moon poised above the smoke, blinking, blinking, as the city is gradually pounded to dust."

Anthony Doerr, *All the Light We Cannot See*

I POSITIONED MYSELF BEFORE MARTHA'S DOOR AND TAPPED GINgerly. Silence loomed. Was she napping? No, not at this hour. I knocked with a bit more resolve and then checked my notes: She had moderate hearing loss and used aids in both ears. So, I delivered a firm wallop to the wood that rattled the door jamb. An eerie stillness hung heavily from the other side, like the calm before a tornado touched down.

I checked my watch three times, a nervous habit, then pushed the door ajar ever so slightly, and announced with trepidation, "Mrs. McCurdy?"

"No one knocks that loudly to attend to my needs. If you must pound the wood into splinters, you don't belong here," she growled. I stepped back.

She added, "I'm tired. Go away."

I was tempted to do just that and document that she refused my visit. Intimidated by her *mug shot,* I was losing my nerve to face her in the flesh. I envisioned her buried under bolts of elephantine tapestry and holding sway amidst important levers and dials in a command post deep within the bowels of an Emerald City-type place.

I peeked around the frame of the door and cleared my throat. She didn't even bother to lift her eyes. A crusty old cop doesn't startle at politeness and subtle overtures of throat-clearing. The room had an elegiac atmosphere.

I stepped across the forbidding threshold.

Martha sat with a walker stationed at her feet. The staff had dressed her portly form in a shapeless, red-and-pink flowered housecoat and planted her upon a cumbrous chair upholstered in a gaudy floral chintz. My first impression of her was one of an uncultivated and uninviting garden. Mustering reserves of courage, I introduced myself.

And out of pure habit, I tacked on my religious moniker, as her granddaughter had precisely instructed me *not* to do. The second it spilled from my lips, I regretted my mistake. Damn. Her sharp mind seized the misstep and sprang into action. Immediately, she swooped in to assess a scheme that might be nefarious to her mind's eye. She unfolded and rose in stages like a sinewy asp swaying to the melody of a snake charmer—all five stocky feet of her—replete with pendulous bosoms swinging. In a matter of seconds, Martha shifted into sergeant mode. The intensity of her mesmerized me.

She propelled herself awkwardly onto the sturdy frame of the walker. Her beady little eyes, perched like a rapt hawk, never left my gaze. It was like she was ready to take a flight from her penthouse aerie. Bony knobs of knuckles enveloped in gnarled veins encircled the metal bars of the walker. Despite her disease and prognosis, she still exuded a modicum of commanding presence from her days on the force. Yet, I moved toward her . . . just in case she needed assistance.

The episode was compelling.

"I have some questions for you . . . chaplain," she spat out with a caustic tone. Her granddaughter had told me that Martha had been mulling insults and allowing wounds to marinate and fester in her mind for years. Up and down, over and under, in and out—existing off the mental scraps of an unresolved trauma—trying to make sense of it all. I understood. It took me years to let go of regrets.

"I have a good one for you," she taunted, hurling years of accumulating venom into one compact lob. Her face flushed red, she got right to the point. "Why does God allow *children* to suffer? And animals?"

And animals. Hmm. She paused while the questions rattled round in my brain like the small metal ball that bounced from target to target in a pinball machine.

"Those kids did nothing wrong. Nothing. Such torment of children is sinful. If God is so powerful and perfect, he should've done something. Kids can't make sense of belts and booze, war, and hunger. They have no status from which to change their predicament or alternatives to pursue. They're just stuck at the mercy of evil."

God was on trial. Therefore, I was on trial for what I represented as a chaplain.

Her room, the size of a child's nursery, was where she now shared her life with the patient in Bed B. That room, with eighty years' worth of odds and ends crammed into the four drawers of an antique dresser was where she called home.

She shifted her stance. I stepped toward her again but only advanced beyond one square of linoleum. After all, a respectful citizen provides a police officer with appropriate space. I was on guard for any physical instability on her part, yet I maintained a deferential distance like I might with a wounded animal.

Martha resumed her dogged pursuit of God's dereliction of duty to safeguard innocence. "Prayer is useless. A waste of time. No one is listening. Believe me, I tried to get that bastard's attention. For hours, I cried . . . silence; for weeks, I pleaded . . . no sign. For months on end, I begged . . . no relief. No navy dropped anchor. No cavalry disembarked. No air force touched down. What could be more precious for God's priorities than children?" Her eyelids fluttered rapidly. I just hoped her heart was not quivering with the same intensity.

Martha focused on the floor, and a string of saliva dribbled down to sprinkle a few flowers on her housecoat. Then she looked up and zeroed in on my eyes like a spike rammed into a stud.

"There is no God."

And there it was—the crowning proclamation declared in the professional and steely manner of a jury delivering a long-sought-after guilty verdict. I envisioned the religious spectators in a packed courtroom erupting in righteous indignation. Her room radiated the heat from searing anger. The lingering heaviness of her impassioned pleas continued to beat down like the unrelenting sun of an August day. I eased her back into the chair.

Dear God. Did she refer to victims from her police work or speak of something equally abhorrent closer to home?

The room was still except for the clock marking time on the bedside table. I hate clocks. I hated the constant ticking of clocks in my home and in the rooms of my patients. No one needed a haughty timekeeper around who counted down the minutes for those in the throes of dying. No one needed a wake-up call for an appointment with the remorseless grim reaper. And no one needed a tenacious tolling of how long one day can truly lag and linger when feeling godforsaken. Human beings already understand that we begin the dying process the day we are born. And then we spend the rest of our lives pretending it isn't true.

I yanked the clock's cord. There. Feeling instantly better, I'd like to think I captured a measure of control as I silenced Father Time. But we both knew it was a dramatic maneuver borne out of frustration and desperation. I was stalling.

Martha, who was flushed with fury, now appeared almost fragile like a withered balloon. When my patients were elderly and gravely ill, time seemed to plod . . . and putter . . . slouch . . . and shuffle . . . and . . . hobble. The flow of time seemed to correspond to age. I plopped myself down onto a folding chair and situated myself off to the side. We both needed a reprieve. And the chill of metal against my damp clothes soothed me for the time being.

We were both battle-weary, but I'd yet to utter a word other than my introduction. My role was to listen and observe. It always amazed me how exhausting that could be, attending so intently to another person. I didn't want to move. I didn't want to talk. My mind was saturated. Martha was my first patient on a list of four, but the others were further along in their spiritual care plans. Thank God. Still, this was going to be a hell of a day.

She cast a sideways glance at me.

Light pierced a crevice in the drawn curtains. I glanced at my watch. Only twenty-five minutes had elapsed since we opened Pandora's Box. Yet, I felt as if I'd been in that stifling room for hours. An aide entered to dispense medications and deal with Martha's personal needs, and I escaped to the hall for a hiatus from the smoldering pile of emotional rubble.

Slumped against the solid surface of Martha's door, the decorative wreath hung at its center encircled my head like a halo. I certainly didn't feel holy. And droplets from a former police officer's indignation had sprayed straight out and into the corridor. A volunteer even coughed as she passed by our door as evidence. After the aide left Martha's room, I knocked on the door again and an impatient voice beckoned. Her voice beckoned? The circumspect tone was as good as a nod in my book, so I sauntered in this time.

In a perfect world, Martha would've waved a little white flag side to side as I entered. Instead, that belligerent thrust of her jaw remained. But less so. Was this subtle change in jaw protuberance only a case of me looking through rose-colored glasses? Apparently, during my baptism by fire in the last hour, I passed some sort of litmus test in her acceptance process.

"You posed good questions. I've voiced that same bewilderment. The same anger." I sat quietly, while she mulled over my genial overture.

"Maybe tomorrow you could tell me the stories of your life that brought you to these questions," I suggested.

Her facial muscles softened, and I saw a twinge of her lower lip. Her talons appeared retracted . . . for now.

Even enraged preschoolers use their fingernails as a defense against threats. But talons also function as part of a deadbolt mechanism: When a key inserts into a lock, it presses down on the metal talon as it's turned and engages the pins to open the door. If the talon breaks, the key can't open the door.

Talons—whether metal or keratin—come in handy during tough times for padlocking hearts or locking out nosy intruders. My role as a chaplain was to find the right key to unlock the door she had shut in everyone's face. Martha had been crying out from the deepest parts of herself with poignant laments. Laments were my favorite psalms. Laments are the prayers of those who are deeply disturbed by the way things are. "Would it be okay for me to visit again?" She didn't say "no." That was progress.

After alerting the staff of my departure, I heaved her chart to my chest, clutched the handle of my rolling suitcase, and trudged down the hall to document our spiritual skirmish. Thick files for other patients occupied the place on the shelf meant for Martha's binder. Thankfully, a social worker from a rival hospice muscled out a chart she needed. As I stuffed Martha into the vacancy, I envisioned crushed flower petals falling from her dress to dust the floor.

I retrieved my credentials from my pocket, flung them around my neck, and took my phone off vibrate to prepare for my next patient. Stepping out of the building, I realized the temperature had plunged at least fifteen degrees. Vestiges of crimson against a cobalt-blue sky greeted me, vibrant and beckoning. The polar opposite of what I left in my wake: spiritless and reticent. A gusty breeze animated the US flag in the courtyard. I inhaled the crisp fragrance of a neighbor's burning leaves and freshly cut grass as if starved for oxygen.

I turned back to glance at Martha's second-floor window. She had legitimate questions that deserved a fair hearing. But old Father Time, iron-fisted and resolute about schedules for the dying, held too many cards. As I got into my car, I remembered an adage that I heard in a theology class: "The heart, like the grape, is prone to delivering its harvest in the same moment that it appears to be crushed." But what if there is nothing to harvest?

Just like Dorothy and her friends learned in *The Wizard of Oz,* Martha did not yet understand that the answers she sought would be found deep within herself. The path to truth always led back home. She appeared crushed, so she might surrender the fruit of her suffering. Time was precious as it filtered through the hourglass, and we had spiritual work to do.

My colleagues would remind me that I shouldn't concern myself if Martha wasn't interested in finding the underlying cause of her bitterness. She was close to dying anyway. What difference would it make? I disagreed. Dying well isn't only about comfort and pain management; it's also about the prospect for spiritual growth until our last dying breath for anyone blessed with a healthy mind.

Richard Rohr asserts, "We are becoming on this side of the door of death, the kind of people we will be on the other side." So I guess life on the other side will be different for each of us. The quality of Martha's eternal life depended on what she planted and harvested on earth. However, the immaturity we might take to our graves does not necessarily mean we're stuck in that stage forever. Therefore, I believe we continue to learn and grow after we die.

On the way to my next patient, I pondered what might be "the key" to unlocking Martha's heart. Martha had envisioned a God (if there was such a being for her) as "a blinking, white cold eye" oblivious to [childhoods] "pounded to dust."

What's in a Name?

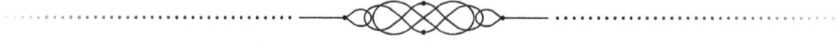

"Everybody needs beauty as well as bread, places to play in and pray in, where nature may heal and give strength to body and mind."

John Muir, Scottish-American naturalist, environmental philosopher, and author

"Wʜᴀᴛ ɪs ʏᴏᴜʀ ɴᴀᴍᴇ ᴀɴᴅ ᴡʜᴀᴛ ᴋɪɴᴅ ᴏғ Gᴏᴅ ᴀʀᴇ ʏᴏᴜ?" That question captured what many of my patients wanted to know as they lay dying. Does God exist? If so, where? How does God exist? What does God do? And for whom and when does God act? In other words, "what's it all about, Alfie?" The Hal David and Burt Bacharach song inspired by the film *Alfie* summed up the meaning of life in 1966, and it's just as pertinent today.

The question about God was from the famous scene in the burning bush narrative. In the book of Exodus (3:1–15), God replied to the question posed by Moses with three words: "ehyeh asher ehyeh." Those three words are so vague that biblical scholars debate their translation, but this phrase is usually rendered, "I Am Who I Am" or "I Will Be What I Will Be." God seemed to evade the question at first glance. But John, Martha, Helen, and George needed to know, and grappled with the nature of God before they died.

When I first read those self-descriptive statements from God in the book of Exodus in a graduate Scripture class, the translations seemed so vague as to be a futile interpretation. God's response to

Moses didn't seem to clarify who God really was. Basically, God said to Moses, "I exist." I could hear Martha guffawing about God's stingy explanation to Moses's logical question about God's identity. For God simply to exist was not good enough for Moses or Martha. A name should inspire us and describe our character like the name Martha chose for her German shepherd, Koda.

Martha suffered abuse during her youth, so her understanding of God was framed by those horrible experiences. She basically described God, "a white cold eye," as author Anthony Doerr described God in *All the Light We Cannot See*. Okay, so Martha finally conceded that God did exist, but then doesn't act. What's the point of worshipping a God who doesn't lift a finger to alleviate suffering? The worst cruelty and evil of all in Martha's book.

Next, God asks Moses to do the impossible: Go to the Pharoah and ask him to release the Israelites. Moses questioned God's judgment. "Who am I, that I should go?" Or: "Yeah, right. I'm not your man. That job is not in my skill set." But God gently responded, "I will be with you." I'm sure Moses was thinking, "You didn't answer my question. And I don't have the qualifications. Aren't there others more fit for the task?" Undeterred, God responded with the utmost patience: "I am with you." God was telling Moses that he could do anything with God's presence and strength.

So, God's name could also be translated as: "I am with you." In Scripture, God gives the name for the Creator as: "I exist" and "I am with you." Again, I can hear Martha's cynical laugh and saying, "Big deal. You exist. But that's the extent of it. You were never with *me*. I didn't see you, feel you, or know you."

However, theologian and biblical scholar Sigmund Mowinckel explains that "the Hebrew verb *hayah/ehyeh* does not mean to *just* exist, but to be active, to express oneself as an active being." The dilemma for most people isn't that a God exists, but how does God exist. That philosophical and theological question was the foundation of my ministry: To help interested patients to figure that out.

Recently, the Gospel passage for Sunday gave another description of God's nature. As the story goes, the Pharisees warned Jesus to leave Jerusalem because Herod had plans to kill him. In response, Jesus called Herod, a "fox." *Jesus had a sly sense of humor.*

In some cultures and folklore, the fox is often portrayed as a trickster: cunning, deceitful, and a symbol of the devil. Two verses later, Jesus used a metaphor to describe himself in reference to the grave threat by foxes as a "hen who gathers her brood under her wings." So, in the Scriptures, God is described as a God who does "exist." Second, God "is always with us." And third, God is like a "Mother Hen."

As a child, I read about hens and foxes—the fox always invaded the chicken coop and caused harm and havoc. And sometimes death. The fox always won. So why would Jesus choose the metaphor of a passive mother hen to describe God? The hen, always at the mercy of the fox, who cannot even keep her chicks safe. I envisioned Martha nodding and saying: *I told you so, chaplain.* And thinking, *Is this for real? God is described as a mother hen who cannot protect her offspring? Even if she wanted to? Wonderful. I've been down that road as a kid, with an incompetent and unloving mother.*

Nadia Bolz-Weber, a Lutheran pastor and author, explains, "A Mother Hen cannot keep a fox from being dangerous . . . but a Mother Hen keeps ravenous foxes (Herod, evil, abuse, suffering, loss, and physical death) from being what determines how we experience the unbelievably beautiful gift of being alive." Even as I write this, I paused here to reflect on this insightful and comforting idea.

God the Creator, the Mother Hen, "gathers all of us under protective wings so that we know where we *belong*. It is there, that we find shelter and love." The pastor goes on to summarize this brilliant Gospel passage, "So in response to our own 'Herods' and to the other very real dangers of this world—our antidotes are compassion, gratitude, forgiveness, kindness, and righteousness."

As a chaplain, I learned that I couldn't fight the "Fox," so I showed my patients how to address the "Foxes" and their own "Herods" in life: childhood abuse, mental health issues, addictions, poor choices, self-sabotage, and victimhood with forgiveness and love. I came to these spiritual realizations over time, as well. God exists. God is always with us. We all belong to God. We are under God's protection against eternal death and for eternal life.

Jesus defied the "Herods" of his life.

Jesus defied death on the wood of an Aspen. A "shield tree."

Jesus gathered Johnny, Martha, Helen, George, and Mark under his wing to turn their deaths into new life.

God desires our safety, wholeness, and spiritual growth.

Martha, does this help you understand what the Creator is? What the creator sees. How the creator acts.

And how does a chaplain help patients who are not Christians come to terms with God and the next world? For example, when I have Native American patients, I utilize their spiritual imagery, literature, art, dance, and cultural rituals. The patient leads the chaplain.

Koda

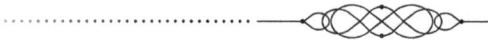

"At his best, man is the noblest of all animals; separated from the law, justice, [and compassion,] he is the worst."

Aristotle, Greek philosopher

THE MORNING DAWNED BRIGHTLY. I FILLED MY COFFEE MUG stamped with a lion and this moniker: "Courage doesn't always roar; sometimes courage is the quiet voice at the end of the day, saying I will try again tomorrow." Often, the quotation on the cup sustained me more than the steaming liquid inside. I grabbed a banana and closed the kitchen door on the noses of two cats.

At the nursing home, I hunted for a vacant space and fetched my small rolling suitcase. I hustled into the lobby to sign in and pumped a glob of gel into my palms. This morning, Martha and I were taking an in-house field trip for my fourth visit. I knocked at her door, which was ajar, announced my presence, and swiftly entered. I hoped my confident stride and momentum might overcome any reluctance on her part. An open door and rays of light greeted me. All hopeful signs. Martha was sitting at the window, an early riser. Her breakfast . . . barely touched.

It was the first time I'd seen the room in full light, and I noticed a pincushion cactus on the windowsill. My elderly aunts always kept cacti around their homes, too. I never understood the fascination with succulents. I always considered them to be prickly, ugly, and boring. My aunts assured me that cacti were valuable, dense with nutrients and medicinal properties. Maybe as we age, like cacti, we collect more barbs, but we also realize the potential for flourishing. Cacti were metaphors for life. I've come to realize that to cherish a cactus, one must reach a certain level of maturity and wisdom in life.

The cactus must receive tender care to blossom, like a child. I had finally grasped the dichotomy of the succulent species: It was both prickly and soft, dormant and fertile, dull and fascinating. Just like human beings. Succulents have shown me that I can grow to be more resilient, multifaceted, fruitful, and beautiful not in spite of challenges, but because of them. I requested a Christmas cactus for my New Year's Eve birthday this year. Now that I'm older, the plant intrigues me. Martha was prickly like a cactus. Her granddaughter was worried about Martha's stern upbringing. I wondered if she had received enough emotional nourishment, tenderness, and love.

After Martha agreed to the in-house mini-retreat, I engaged the brakes to stabilize the wheelchair and helped her get into it. We were on our way. Not surprisingly, my pace quickened to match the spirited activity of the unit. I rambled on about nothing of consequence until I thought to ask her why she had a cactus. Martha didn't respond.

Our moods shifted as we approached the small chapel in the west wing. It was otherworldly in that intimate space . . . sacred, silent, and serious. It demanded reverence, respect, and truth from its visitors. I posted the "In Use" sign at the entrance. It had a pithy saying tacked below it: "The struggle is real, but so is God."

My anxiety settled, and I spoke in hushed tones. Light streaming through the stained glass illuminated stories of Christ. Scanning the windows, I recognized a familiar scene of Jesus in a fishing boat with his disciples; it portrayed the calming of the waters from Mark's gospel.

Encouraged, I asked a weary-looking Martha where I should position her and then pulled up my chair. We sat in silence. My soul soaked up the serenity of the space. Martha's eyes were closed. Suddenly she opened them and sat as straight as a ramrod. She stared at the small altar and the crucifix hanging above it. One hand rested on each thigh, her gnarled fingers splayed as if she were preparing to testify in a court proceeding for her precinct.

"I still remember that morning," she began. "Overcast and damp, it was. Before breakfast, my mother marched us out back in single file just as we were ushered into Mass every Sunday. 'Look, here come those well-behaved Jozwiak children.' I'm sure that's what parishioners whispered."

I hadn't prompted her. It was like a reporter pressed "record" on a camera, and she relished the opportunity to set the record straight.

"I will never forget the sound of the coiled rope scraping against the scales of the bark on our oak," Martha went on. "My German shepherd, Koda, was swinging frantically and straining the outstretched limb. He struggled to free himself from the grasp of the noose. His eyes bore down on mine, pleading for mercy and confused by this quick turn of events in his life. We stood frozen; all *five* of us—in a row, a ragtag group we were. My two sisters and two brothers. We just stood there—stunned. The color drained from our faces as Koda's big, brown eyes rolled back and his muscular body went limp."

I reached for Martha, but she raised her hand as if to say, let me finish. Now I understood. Her anger. The bitterness. And cynicism. The prickly nature.

She paused and looked down at her lap, picking at the loose threads of the blanket. I was barely breathing, stunned by the unfolding story. The steely demeanor she had acquired over all those years was evident in this room. "My nine-year-old brother, Tom, vomited. Cassie whimpered and squeezed my hand. I never got a good look at Billy's face. The littlest one, Meg, continued to wet our bed for months. I oversaw her laundry so our mother wouldn't notice."

I was dazed, bereft of emotion. Luckily, she wasn't soliciting comfort.

Martha recounted the sickening scene: "The corpse swayed back and forth—the rope creaked and strained under his dead weight. Oddly, I remembered our tire swing rotated in the opposite direction beneath him, creating the most morbid dance between the two."

Anger swelled within me, but I maintained an outward calm—barely.

"How did it come to that?"

"My mother was the instigator. I'm sure about that. She stood there, near the tree, with a look of glassy-eyed satisfaction. I watched a smug smile creep across her face. She was a crazy bitch. The ladder that my parents used to hoist Koda leaned against the shed. She would've needed help, so I had no illusions that my old man wasn't involved, but he was nowhere to be seen. I'm sure they shared a pint of whiskey over their eggs before they strung Koda up."

What came next sounded like the thin, high-pitched, and plaintive voice of a young girl.

"I was eleven years old; Koda was six. He slept in my bed when my mother wasn't around. When we got him, I looked up dog names: The word Koda means 'ally' or 'friend' in the Sioux language. He was all of that and more."

Then the monologue halted. She shifted in the chair and moved her hands from her lap to the armrests and clutched each one. Horrified, I offered her water. And a Kleenex. I had heard many unfortunate stories as a chaplain, but this was obscene.

Suddenly, I felt transported to their dank backyard, where the children had stood overwhelmed by grief. We stood frozen on the lawn—all *six* of us now—nauseated and numb. We wanted to scream in protest, but our throats were parched. The freezing rain and our anguish soaked us to the bone. It was then I recalled Rabbi Kushner's insightful theology about how God suffers with us. So, I presumed we were now *seven* standing in that row. Shivering, shaking, sobbing. We huddled together in the solidarity of sorrow and shock.

At last, my voice unleashed a guttural tone I didn't recognize. It sounded otherworldly even to my own ears. And then Martha's tone adopted a sing-song quality.

"Koda hung there for most of the morning, twisting in the wind and rain—a constant reminder that any mistakes would be punished swiftly for anyone unfortunate enough to belong to our household. My siblings and I always stood with the sword of Damocles poised over us, its steel blade dangling by the breadth of a whisker."

"How were you punished?" I thought of Kat's earlier comments.

"We got the belt for tardiness, laziness, and mouthing off. And me? For neglecting to wipe the dust from the top of the door frames. That was my job. I couldn't even reach the top of the door frame. No one dusts there."

"What was Koda's sin?"

"Apparently, he soiled her good rug. He must've eaten something rotten."

She turned to me and blurted, "I hated her. I still hate her. She was no 'mother hen.'"

The cross hanging at the front of the chapel looked bulkier now, as if it had gained fifty pounds transferring to itself Martha's substantial list of parental transgressions. I thought of the aspen trees from the day on the lake. According to Christian mythology, the leaves of the poor poplar tree tremble in shame forever because its trunk supplied the wood for the cross.

Martha cocked her head toward the door. She had said what she came to say.

I knelt before her as I unlocked the brakes on either side of the chair. I looked straight into her milky-blue eyes. The tears were a hopeful sign. I remembered the psalm that comforted me during my own trials and recited it to her.

"Save me, God. I am in floodwater, and the water is up to my neck. Deeper and deeper, I have sunk into the mire. I can't find a stronghold to stand on. I'm exhausted from crying out for help, and my throat is parched. I am distressed. My sight blurs because of my tears. My body and soul are wasting away. I am dying from grief; my years are shortened by sadness."

"That's exactly how I feel," she said. "That's in the Bible?"

I nodded. "Psalm 69. Hebrew scriptures."

Reaching for her hands, I continued. "It was written around twenty-five hundred years ago." Feeling "stuck in the mire" and yelling for help in "neck-deep, rising flood water" appears to be a universal situation and emotion no matter what era one lived in.

"We are so much more than our grim stories, Martha. We have to be. God was inconsolable, witnessing the abuse you endured." I thought about another patient of mine who had survived a Nazi concentration camp.

Martha clutched her wadded-up tissue. "*God* was inconsolable? God's *sorrow* doesn't protect children and animals from horror. I don't really care that God was inconsolable. How does that work exactly? God should be the primary custodian of safety and goodness. Isn't that right, chaplain?"

My well-meaning guidance was greeted with derision.

"You spend your days peddling that pathetic crap to the most vulnerable of people—the sick, the oldest of the elderly, and the suffering."

Her eyes were hard. What opposition could I muster? I had a mostly idyllic childhood.

But, as I look back, God didn't remove my trials any more than those of others but supported my courage and hope. God provided me with unforeseen circumstances and opportunities to develop certain strengths, virtues, values, and faith to prepare me for whatever might come my way in a harsh world. As a first-born, I had forged a resiliency, a formidable personality, an independent spirit, critical thinking, and a resolve to plow through life's obstacles that hindered God's path for me. CS Lewis also said: "It doesn't do any good to move forward on the wrong road."

How does one know the right road? One must slow down and pay attention to the details and circumstances of life. Ask for signs and a navigable path. Live in the present moment. In other words, it's what mystics call becoming conscious. For me, I started being more conscious in my late forties.

The surgery I needed for a bowel obstruction forced me to pursue a path that I never would've taken on my own. Sadly, my anesthesiologist failed to examine my throat before surgery and tried to jam the wrong-sized intubation equipment down my larynx. In the process, he damaged my vocal cords. If you remember, I had a degree in vocal music and the physician's negligence that morning ended my capability to perform, sing for weddings, funerals, or audition to sing in semi-professional community choruses. Singing and acting was the way I expressed myself as a wife, mother, teacher, and chaplain. Today, I cannot sustain a decent phrase and my upper range has been seriously compromised. But on the spectrum of victimization in this world, I got off easy.

But God knew better. I had eventually come to realize that the surgical miscue that morning had forced me to follow an alternate path—a path of pastoral counselling, hospice work, speaking, and writing. And the same for Mark's life. When he was airlifted to Gundersen Lutheran Hospital, the thoracic surgeon said that Mark had a one percent chance of making it out of the stream that February day, back to his car, and transported to a major trauma center for triple-bypass surgery.

That extra time God provided Mark to continue living was redemptive for both of us. We needed to attend to some personal issues and marital problems that had cropped up. But we didn't understand the significance of that precious statistic at the time.

I explained to Martha that it inspired me how she managed an abusive childhood, mothered her siblings, had handled a teen pregnancy, single parenting, and the premature deaths of her husband and only daughter, yet achieved an impressive career in law enforcement.

"What did you make of that? Did you take the time to look back? To connect all of the dots?"

Martha was staring at me. I could see the realizations surfacing on her face.

"You didn't accomplish those milestones on your own. Something certainly sustained you."

Using the arms of Martha's chair to pull myself up from the floor, I felt the stiffness in my fifty-eight-year-old body. I swung her toward the door, and my eyes swept over the beaten body of Christ hanging from the wood of the aspen at the front of the chapel. The limp image of Koda swinging from the branch of an oak came to mind.

"The Spirit of Christ was never oblivious to your trials. The Breath of Life saw you, knew you, and loved you." I flipped the chapel sign back to "unoccupied" for the next soul, and we retraced our steps back to her room, each lost in our thoughts.

Water, Wind, and Gulls

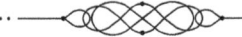

"Right now, the shadows of clouds are dragging across the water, and patches of sunlight are touching down everywhere. White strings of gulls drag over it like beads."

Anthony Doerr, All the Light We Cannot See

I CHECKED THE STRAPS SECURING MY THIRTEEN-FOOT KAYAK TO the saddles on top of my car—still snug. I threw an overnight bag into the back seat amidst paddles, a life vest, and a canvas tote full of groceries. I did not relish the three-hour drive north navigating miles of concrete and construction barrels with rush-hour drivers and weekend traffic. But I'd reap the rewards awaiting me in Door County (known as the Cape Cod of the Midwest) and a generous three-day reprieve from dying patients and their emotional and spiritual issues.

I was driving to the Torinus summer place, called the "Omelet." My husband's grandparents named it when they built the sprawling structure in Egg Harbor, Wisconsin, in the 1930s. My children did not want to stray from the "egg" theme when the opportunity to christen our speed boat presented itself, so "Sunnyside Up" spent the 1990s moored at the city dock.

The name Door County originated from the Potawatomi tribe whose hundreds of members drowned trying to cross the chief navigational passage at the tip of the peninsula between the Bay of Green Bay and Lake Michigan. So, the Potawatomi coined that passage, "the Door of Death." To this day, in bad weather, the roiling waves of both bodies of water merge at that tip and create a fierce undertow.

Aware of the legend, our family and guests felt comfortable navigating the vortex above watery graves on a car ferry on our trips farther north to Washington Island. I always seemed to find myself at the doorway to some type of demise in my life. According to guides about astrological signs, that is a typical experience of those born under the sign of Capricorn.

I relished some alone time for a weekend, as Mark joined a good friend for a short, easy hunt for pheasants on Saturday. A month had passed since a staph infection had invaded Mark's pacemaker leads, and during the surgery to replace them, the cardiac surgeons needed to place him on a ventilator for a week to relieve the additional burden on his heart. After a few strenuous weeks of hospice work and then bedding down in a rigid hospital recliner for three days next to Mark, I needed time to reboot and get refreshed.

I maneuvered through a snarl of drivers snaking their way toward exit ramps of the bedroom communities and suburbs that stretched far beyond Milwaukee, my mind still in total hospice mode. I had been thinking a lot about Martha's spiritual care plan, wondering how I could ease the resentment that had festered in her mind for decades.

Soon, the pastoral scenery of the countryside replaced the suburban sprawl of malls and car dealerships, and the knots in my neck loosened. But it took until the village of Luxemburg to overcome my preoccupation with Martha. I stopped to buy fresh cheese curds at a roadside market and a soft-serve vanilla cone at the Frosty Tip to celebrate.

Now, alternating rows of golden wheat and barley shimmered in the breeze alongside crops of vivid green the farther north I traveled. I enjoyed the checkered pattern they created—precise and predictable, so unlike my life. Shabby, crimson barns bent under their own lopsided weight, livestock foraging through dusty fields for grain, and cement silos brimming with silage peppered the hilly landscape. The quaint vista was marred only by the occasional roadside billboard promoting the autumn tourist attractions.

Classical vocal music helped absorb the miles of the long road trip, and I entered the outskirts of Egg Harbor by dusk, earlier than planned. As I turned onto the road to my destination, I approached the grove of stately birch that stood sentry for almost a century at the obscure entrance of our summer place. The stone wall enclosing the property separated the two-acre parcel from adjacent neighbors. Golden rod and brown-eyed Susan carpeted the forest floor on both sides of the driveway. I guided my car over the exposed, gnarly tree roots that protruded through the gravel-packed dirt.

In the circular drive at the back entrance, I opened my driver's side door and was flooded with the fragrance of cedar and the deep purple of its berries dangling from slender sleeves of emerald leaves. Inhaling the sweet scent, I plucked a finger of its bent offering. I shed my sandals to the moss-covered path as I approached the front of the property. The view always brought me to a standstill, each gull screeching and swooping, their squalling cries welcomed me to this time-worn sanctuary.

The bay camouflaged itself as a fresh-water ocean, an aqueous surface as far as the eye could see, nestled between two fingers of land. On stormy days, twelve-foot waves devoured the dock. It was often either beauty or beast in its temperament.

The scent of algae and mossy seaweed filled my nostrils. For miles, the bay stretched—clear, calm, and sparkling, its expanse undisturbed except for the occasional island or iron-ore freighter dotting the horizon. I made a quick inspection through our imposing structure and grabbed a beach towel. There were believable rumors that Great-Aunt Bertha still roamed the dark halls of the second floor, so I threw my belongings in the master bedroom on the first floor so as not to provoke her restless spirit.

My door had a lock that was useless to her spectral form, but I figured she would respect my need for serenity. And privacy. After all, she wasn't some random ghost wandering the halls to perturb, but a beloved ancestor whose passed-down piece of furniture, known as The Secretary, stood stately in our home office. I treasured that antique and took special care of it. *Bertha, are you listening?*

Soon, the outdoor shower enticed me, and I dropped my clothes to the planks of its knotty pine deck. Threads of grass tickled my toes through the slats below. Warm water poured from the spout, cleansing my mind, rinsing the previous week of work down the drain.

No boats were passing, and the cabins nearby were already winterized and shuttered, so I went out toward the rocky shore and allowed the light breeze to caress my naked body and mind. The setting sun saturated the evening sky, and its bouquet of coppery colors encircled my outstretched arms. I twirled in the freedom of it all. A dance of delight. A celebration of joy. Pure ecstasy.

Wildly, I cavorted in the company of Sister Moon, flitting gulls, and gusts of wind. Bowing and bending. Sashaying and swirling. Hospice protocols, policies, and palliative-care plans had evaporated thanks to the stunning diversion of what lay before me. Slipping into the shadowy silhouettes of the inky inlet, I immersed myself in its fortifying grace and absolution. Frolicking and floating in the darkness, my concerns dissolved one by one as each new star broke through the mantle of clouds that obscured the breadth of heaven.

I slept well that night. Two full days and nights to release my responsibilities and take care of myself—to concentrate on my body and *my soul,* for once.

The slender peninsula that separated the eastern edge of the state from Lake Michigan was like a treasure chest filled with antidotes for a chaplain's weary spirit. In that place, I soaked my soul in glistening water, and kayaked through dark sea caves teeming with blowholes and bats. In that place, I delighted in folklore theater under luminous skies and the watchful eyes of hooting owls. In that place, I hiked limestone cliffs and climbed rickety ladders only to disappear into the crowns of leafy branches bursting with honey crisp apples. My bucket brimming with near-perfect specimens of crunchy sweetness.

Mark and I had savored the religious retreats on the grounds of Chambers Island. I tittered through the first dinner and breakfast unaccustomed to the imposed silence, and therefore the lack of noisy camaraderie at the large circular tables set for eight. But I came to appreciate the round-the-clock serenity and space it created for contemplation.

Mark was an experienced sailor and acquainted with the hazards of each harbor and the isolated islands that buffered miles of cliffs. Like pearls, the small islands were strung like beads, parallel to the peninsula. Our small skiff skimmed the tops off frothy waves as he navigated in and out of dangerous shoals and shallow sandbars. I trusted him in everything.

But then it was Sunday. It always arrived too quickly. I tidied up, gathered my belongings, and bid farewell to Aunt Bertha. As I looked around the place one last time, a multitude of memories flooded over me of Mark, our three children, the first grandchild, and the succession of four hunting dogs fetching Frisbees off the dock. We had summered there for forty years, often with relatives and friends in tow. I was jealous of the gulls who never packed a suitcase to leave this place or of the necessity to return to a demanding career.

Mark's older brother, Tom, who died in 2021, wrote of this scenic view from the stoop of the Omelet: "Do not think the white gull wheeling over these breaking waves has found freedom. She is a slave to the scene. Your kind of freedom she does not want, for she has chosen, and she has been chosen. Long after you have moved on, she will hover here in constant love. She will never leave the heaving breast of this breathing bay."

For two weeks at a stretch, our family explored acres of bluffs and swales, cliffs and caves, estuaries and orchards, and the exquisite galleries of acrylics and watercolors that forever captured a scene we couldn't live without. I wasn't ready to leave. I never was. I wanted to be "a slave to that scene, and cleave to that heaving breast." That breast of spiritual nourishment that was, The Bay. I wanted to be that gull that "hovered in constant awe" and staked its claim for a parcel of this view. Yes, I wanted "to possess the freedom of the gull," for far longer than a week's stay.

But my existence was attached to a different place and choice. My role was to give my patients the wings to fly free of this world—to prepare them to die well. But though my weekend with the gulls always left me with some regret, their scenic presence created a healthier and more compassionate chaplain.

After I packed my car, my sight was focused on death once again.

Nature of the Divine

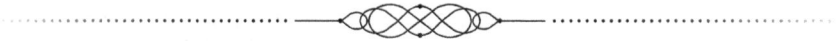

"If I take one step at a time, I have just enough light for the step I'm on."

S. Omartian, Christian author

As I drove home, I reflected on how Martha had tried to barter with God for years, but then concluded that a God didn't exist. No Ultimate Source. No Divine Light. No Eternal Being of Unconditional Love. Nothing. She was bursting with anger. But at whom? Beneath it all, I suspected that Martha did believe in something greater than herself or why bother with such self-depleting ire.

As a chaplain, sometimes I was in the position to correct misconceptions about God; and in the process, I was in fact rectifying the patient's negative beliefs about themselves and their situations. Distorted beliefs about God and reality can keep a person stuck in anxiety, depression, and religiosity which can lead to cynicism or self-righteousness.

One of my favorite theologians was St. Catherine, who lived in Siena, Italy, in the fourteenth century. Mark and I had visited her birthplace. As a mystic, she attained such a deep relationship with God that she possessed knowledge that no one else had achieved. So, what did Catherine know that priests, popes, and monks didn't? Could that wise woman of the 1300s reach across centuries to help me with Martha?

Two hours into the drive home, a familiar tightness crawled back into my shoulders and climbed upward, burrowing deep in its favorite spot, my neck. I searched for an exit with a gas pump and a convenience store to stretch, and when I spotted one, I bought a prepackaged turkey sandwich, chips, and a diet soda.

As I settled back in for the long drive, I remembered Catherine's theological insight into the nature of God. She wrote, "Strange that so much suffering is caused because of the misunderstanding of God's true nature." So, the world would endure less suffering if we just understood God better? It took until my seventeenth year in Catholic education during my religious studies graduate program in natural theology to get a grip on the nature of God.

Catherine went on to describe an element of God's ultimate nature. "God's heart is gentler than Mary's first kiss upon Jesus." I thought about my first grandchild, James. Ten minutes after his birth, I cradled his precious body and watched the tears streaming down the unshaven and exhausted face of my son. Never will I forget that first, gentle kiss upon my grandson's sweet lips and the searing love for him that caught my breath.

Finally, I understood how God had always felt about me. About everyone. And I grasped how God could possess the gentlest of hearts and love us to pieces and still not swoop into our lives like the cavalry every time we suffered. Catherine knew firsthand what suffering entailed because she spent her life working with the poor, the oppressed, and the sick. She died at thirty-three after paralysis struck her lower body and a severe stroke managed to cripple the rest of her. Incidentally, I assumed Catherine was a Capricorn.

Martha's perception of God didn't square with Catherine's notion. If God's heart was so gentle, merciful, and caring, how did that all-encompassing love reconcile the tremendous suffering in the world? As I understood it, God was either loving and merciful to everyone, or God was not loving and merciful at all. I had experienced enough love and mercy from God to know deep in my gut which was true.

Catherine wrote, "We all suffer more because of our unreasonable expectations for what God's love and mercy can accomplish for us on earth." Or, to put it bluntly, God's mercy and love doesn't promise an around-the-clock rescue service. But miracles do happen. Large and small. So, who receives the divine intervention? It's a mystery.

When I was a younger woman, I interpreted God's nature to be a safety net. I mistook my white privilege for blessings bestowed by the Creator. How naïve. I falsely believed that if I was a good person, followed the "rules," worked hard, and "prayed" fervently, God was at my beck and call. I found out it didn't work that way. Nor should it.

Love and justice are the antidotes for problems in the world. However, watching the evening news of the war in Ukraine, witnessing the terror and oppression of German citizens living on the wrong side of the Berlin Wall in 1973, and seeing photos of the bodies of Syrian children in 2015—victims of immigration gone awry—washed up on the shores of Greece and Turkey was a quick reminder that humans must respond to the inequities in the world. But it seems as if the reserves of compassion and large-scale resources in the world pale in the presence of God's perfect capabilities.

Why shouldn't God be the first responder and we, the benchwarmers, could go in as backup? I grappled with the same angry questions as Martha: *"Where the hell was God amidst it all?"*

Eventually, I learned to see where God was present in my life despite the periods of emotional suffering and physical pain, but the process took me into my early fifties to sort it all out. My role was to help Martha recognize God's loving activity in her life amidst the abuse. We are all at different stages in sorting all of this out, but the key is to keep trying.

I remember the exact day I came to spiritual adulthood—in the manner of the iconic question, "Where were you when the Twin Towers collapsed?" Those of us in the United States will always remember where we were on September 11, 2001, at 8:46:40 a.m. EST. On the day thousands of innocent Americans died, I was driving to teach high school students about the difference between morality and ethics. All I had to do that morning was to turn on the television for a ready-made lesson plan and discussion.

It was an ordinary day when I received my stroke of insight. After clearing the dinner dishes from the table, I hunkered down with a glass of Zin to read and I stumbled across an existential theory by a popular Jewish theologian, Rabbi Harold Kushner. It was August 20, 2005, at 7:30 p.m. CST. And then I read this: "God is all-powerful, but God's power does not include the capacity to reverse the evil consequences stemming from 'free will.' God's love for us neither avoids nor invades the soul's suffering. It is a love that does not 'fix' us but gives us strength by suffering with us."

What? Stunned, I reread his solemn statement over and over. Initially, it was not a comforting discovery. "What good did it do to suffer *with* someone?" Kushner's keen observation and knowledge hurled me into a vault of vulnerability that I'd never felt before, like that of a forsaken orphan or stray dog combing alleys for edible garbage.

God does not protect us from the travails of this world, but God does sustain us through them; the "Mother-hen theology." I didn't want this fact to be true.

Children could not escape the negative consequences of others' misguided decisions, either. Like Martha, I didn't want God to suffer *with* me; I wanted God to *end* my suffering. I hadn't yet made the correlation between the concepts of unconditional love, freedom, and dignity. It made sense now. Free will was a precious gift with a huge price tag. God's nature prevented God from eliminating the consequences of humanity's horrible choices. The result? God often came across as an impersonal bystander to our suffering and blunders.

Perhaps St. Catherine was trying to say that we reach spiritual adulthood when we can accept God's authentic nature and the realities of our own lives. Then, we ultimately grow up.

Finally, I reached the western suburbs of Milwaukee, and the musing came to an end. The shores of Lake Michigan had kept my ministry at bay for three precious days. I pulled out my work cell and listened to the hospice report line from the weekend. The on-call nursing staff updated admissions and deaths every morning and evening. So, I was back in the saddle.

After unpacking the car, I slipped into my pjs, scooped strawberry ice cream into a cereal bowl, and gathered the cats onto my lap to watch a mindless movie while I waited for Mark to come home. As we were getting ready for sleep, I thanked God for my hubby at my side, "The Omelet," and the beauty of the Peninsula. I basked in the glow of that spiritual weekend until my eyelids grew heavy.

Helen

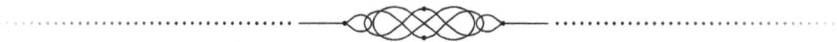

"You must have a strong foundation when the winds of change shift."

Bob Dylan, singer, songwriter, author, visual artist

It was Monday. On my way to my next patient after visiting Martha, I was belting out tunes from an ABBA soundtrack when our nursing administrator called. She wanted me to check in before I continued with my afternoon appointments.

Apparently, my sixty-year-old patient Helen was spending her last hours on our service. Live discharges do happen in the hospice world. Normally, that would be a positive turn of events for everyone involved. However, in this case, it was the legal thing to do but not the moral one. Removing her eleven months ago would've been the legal and moral thing to do.

I had broached the topic concerning her length of stay at medical meetings, but without success. Now, our administrator was dispatching me to oust Helen from our service. Unlike our two former physicians, our new medical director was alarmed at the length of her "residency" with our company. My task was to bring the paperwork to her, get it signed, and hightail it back.

My patient had been under our care for more than a year. During those months, her medical diagnosis seemed irrelevant to our company. No one should reside in hospice as long as Helen; it raised red flags. To be eligible for hospice, a patient must have a terminal diagnosis and a prognosis of dying within six months. It was clear from the beginning that Helen had neither qualification. National statistics showed that the average person remained on a hospice service for about three weeks. This was not an enviable statistic either. The Medicare benefit gives end-of-life care for six months. Most people do not take advantage of the generous time frame.

Helen genuinely believed that she was dying, regardless of medical evidence that proved otherwise. She suffered from a chronic and painful condition, but she was not dying. A more appropriate placement for Helen would've been inpatient treatment with a hospice company certified to care for those with chronic illnesses in a palliative care setting. However, Medicare does not reimburse hospice companies as handsomely for palliative care costs so we have less resources to offer chronically ill patients who suffer but are not dying.

I had been visiting her weekly since the fall of 2011. When our two former medical directors departed from the company, the physician who replaced them examined our documentation for each patient and booted those he considered inappropriate for hospice. It was clear our agency needed to act with urgency because state auditors were arriving soon to review our books.

Eventually, our company had garnered the attention of the Centers for Medicare and Medicaid Services and its contractors for questionable admissions, and we were being probed for incomplete claims submitted for reimbursement of patient care. We hired a full-time (in-house) RN just to address all of our patient claims. This RN position was not one you'd want to advertise publicly.

CMS required additional documentation when a company couldn't properly settle a patient Medicare claim. These requests were not standard protocol when hospice providers documented correctly, were not negligent, and were ethical about admissions and discharges. Sometimes families balked at the removal of loved ones from our service, but hospice was not free adult daycare. Dying in a timely manner was a prerequisite, unfortunately.

Helen had no idea of the doom about to descend upon her. She had used the levels of morphine we prescribed to her for chronic pain. Her husband lived on the East Coast, and other family members were scattered throughout the Midwest. Our hospice had become like an adoptive family for her, so when her long nights lingered and loneliness prevailed, she became a regular patron for our third-shift answering service and its on-call RN. And she was chatty.

Helen recited the rosary daily, and Mother Angelica's weekly religious lectures on cable television captivated her. She looked forward to my visits for receiving Communion. For every appointment, she insisted we prepare her soul as if it were her last day on earth. It always surprised and disappointed Helen that her "last day" never arrived. Circled calendar dates for "the day of dying" came and went, so Helen hunkered down in Room 122, content with her routine of morphine, lorazepam, and arts and crafts projects. But Helen was no milquetoast; she was cocky and tenacious. I called her Chief.

My suspicion about her long tenure on hospice was that we'd gotten her addicted to morphine, and we didn't know what else to do with her. She was not my only patient who had taken advantage of our service to discreetly subsidize a drug addiction. It wasn't prevalent, so we ignored it.

Helen descended upon our agency one blustery day as a faceless statistic during one of those patient-roundup contests we held twice a year. I got to know Helen well from our jaunts to her favorite neighborhood restaurant for the all-you-can-eat pancake special each Tuesday. She navigated her motorized wheelchair around bumps in the roadway like a seasoned racecar driver, often with me chasing her. Crucial evidence that death was not sitting on her doorstep.

Helen had no inkling that her trustworthy and loyal chaplain, of all people, was about to dispense with her. My greatest worry was that our RN hadn't warned Helen's primary care doctor about this abrupt departure and neither of them had fair notice that our morphine pipeline was about to dribble to nothing. I called members of our clinical team during my drive there.

Compassion had always been at the root of our company mission. As a patient, Helen was a stakeholder in our company; she had a personal stake in the clinical decisions that affected her. The timing of this discharge was unprofessional and conducted without an ounce of kindness. But an emphasis on a singular bottom line to generate wealth was not exactly a breeding ground for integrity.

After taking the longest route to the facility I could find, I arrived in forty-five minutes to the sprawling one-story structure with blue shutters. I resumed stalling once inside. I signed in. Pumped a splat of disinfectant. Looked for the loo. Followed the floor manager to her office to chat, poured a cup of caffeine, and hunted down the powdered creamer. Then I nibbled on one of my chipped nails in the unoccupied chapel and fervently prayed that Helen would somehow be out of the building. My unwelcome assignment was to pull the floor out from under my patient with nothing but a dark, forlorn cellar full of cobwebs and drained medical vials to replace it.

I surveyed the participants in the activity room and glimpsed Helen's funky maxi dress, matching flowered headband, and suede fringe-infested vest, all in different shades of vivid purple and pink. She noticed my presence and beckoned me forward. As I slid out a chair next to her, she yelled, "BINGO!" The volume startled me.

While she examined the basket of prize-winning goodies and claimed her reward, I clamped down on the handles of her wheelchair and steered toward the private lounge. She cradled the bottle of lilac-scented body wash in her lap like a seven-year-old birthday recipient and chattered all the way down the hall.

I tried to explain "the problem," stammering and skimming over the abrupt and looming departure. Why didn't they send the RN case manager for such a delicate "political" maneuver that pertained to her health-care? She was the medical expert. Whenever management had a sticky problem, they outsourced a chaplain. I guess they calculated that having God somewhere in the equation would make the bitter medicine go down easier. But that is not how it works.

She looked flustered and frightened all at once. I couldn't blame her. Helen understood the implications of this unscheduled visit—she wasn't dying after all and worse, there would be no more morphine. Or anything else. We went step by step through the discharge paperwork, and she signed on the dotted line marked with an X in glaring red ink.

Our administrator also made sure to specify the exact spot by surrounding the dotted line with a bold black box—daring Helen to miss the red bull's eye—which further highlighted the weight of her signature. The emblazoned box felt like the garrote dangling from a hillside gallows as the victim shuffled toward it.

Did Helen really understand the ramifications of that one stroke of her pen? That her anemic scrawl would excise a solid team of professionals from her daily and weekly routine? Her RN, social worker, chaplain, and certified nursing assistant would never be able to visit again. Hugging her, I recited one of her favorite prayers. Then, I thought to bestow a final blessing. Her favorite hymn came to mind.

Chaplain, you cannot preach, pray, explain, sing, or bless your way out of this mess.

We returned to Room 122, both of us moping. I tried to raise additional and rational explanations for her plight, but we both knew that there were none. I got her settled in front of Mother Angelica and replaced the bottle of body wash in her lap with a strand of crystal rosary beads strapped to her fingers. Everything I offered to soothe her soul was superficial and inadequate, like putting a Band-Aid on a stab wound. She would continue to reside at the facility, but nothing could minimize the pain of such a blunt excision from our medical services. I knew Helen would be in a constant state of brooding and anxiety about this huge medical, social, and emotional upheaval.

Before I left, I gave Helen a grounding figurine. A smooth wooden angel. Like a grounding stone, it fit in the palm of her hand, and I hoped it would help her feel connected to a physical reality when she felt panicked and unmoored. I had told her to keep the blessed figurine in her pocket and to hold it when she was afraid. Often, I had purchased sacred medals or small statutes to give to my patients and students when they needed a tangible reminder that they were going to be okay when no other emotional support was available. She nodded when I said that I would pray for her.

Yes, Helen had survived hospice. Most people would say she had dodged a bullet. But she didn't want to dodge death. She wasn't afraid to die. She was perpetually ready and simply marking time. On a *shortcut* back to the office, which took all of twenty minutes, I rehearsed the speech I planned to unload on my administrator. The slide in our service continued to annoy me, but the thought of quitting my job was not an option. I was the main breadwinner, carried our health insurance, and we had bills to pay. Not to mention that Mark had a three-year prognosis without a transplant, and we were zeroing on that dreaded date.

Soon, I sat before the formidable desk of our administrative RN and launched into the details of our dereliction on behalf of Helen, for other patients, and the treatment of employees. Sporting the Mona Lisa smile, Yvonne thanked me for my concern, rose to open the door, and showed me out. She kicked me to the curb with a flourish of her hand, not interested in addressing my concerns—at least not in my presence. This type of patient discharge hadn't been anywhere near standard protocol when I started working at Hospice Advantage.

I never saw Helen again, and then, one day, *three years later*, I noticed her obituary. I was one of those hospice chaplains who combed through the weekly death announcements. At the funeral, I peered into the casket, and, yes, it really was the Chief. My Helen. She had managed to die. Finally. She wore a mask of contentment and the linen dress she had chosen just for this occasion. And nestled securely in her folded hands was the wooden figurine. I touched her cheek. That was the day I stopped praying for her.

She had been *escorted* home.

As I walked out of the church, I remembered the words of the founder of the first modern hospice, Cicely Saunders: *"We will help you live well until you die."*

Contributing to a patient's drug addiction is not helping a person "live well." And keeping a patient on hospice service when death is four years away from the initial admission is incompetent, unethical, and illegal.

Visions and Signs

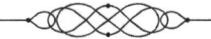

"Life is amazing. And then it's awful. And then it's amazing again. And in between the amazing and the awful, it's ordinary, mundane, and routine ... breathe in the amazing and hold on through the awful. That's just living. And it's breathtakingly beautiful."

LR Knost, award-winning author, feminist, social justice activist, and founder of a children's rights advocacy and family consulting group.

MY WEEK BEGAN WITH A VISIT TO THE FIRST-FLOOR LOUNGE that had a lovely view of the grounds. Vibrant mums in shades of yellow, purple, and crimson brightened the patio along with cornstalks, pumpkins, and bales of hay. A scarecrow bolstered a pole of flickering gaslight.

I snatched two Halloween cookies and fetched two mugs of cider from the kitchen. My mission this day was to find out how Martha was coping after divulging the reams of resentments, regrets, and trauma of her battered youth. She had bemoaned the loss of her companion, Koda. A chaplain can only help so much; I'm not a psychologist, and neither was our social worker.

We settled near a bay window overlooking an outdoor feeder that entertained residents and guests with the fluttering and fidgeting of a variety of feathered species. Nuthatches, chickadees, and wrens were grabbing breakfast and ferrying seeds to nests tucked beneath the eaves and hidden amidst dense pine branches. I set a cassette on the table and asked Martha if I could record our conversation. She shrugged.

I inserted the tape and pressed "record." We began gingerly—musing about the antics of birds, our favorite seasons, and what we were most grateful for. Martha mentioned her deceased husband, Kat, and Ladybug. Listening to the tales of her formidable career, I asked what legacy she was most proud of.

She took time to consider her own broad footprint: "I tried to salvage the childhoods of my siblings with diversion . . . silly jokes, nature walks, art projects, and affection—trying to saturate their souls with the security and innocence that our parents had robbed from each of them. I did the best I could. As they got older, I tried to protect them from the world outside of our house before I left. Not that it was any worse than what they had experienced inside our home."

"Hmm. Protect them. Were you able to 'protect' them out there, on their own, in our wounded world?"

"Not very well. It was tough watching them make serious mistakes and stumble. But I tried to be available to support and guide them. They knew how much I loved them."

"That sounds like the same dilemma and heartache that God experiences with us." I hoped Martha had caught the correlation between her caretaking and that of God.

We watched a junco and sparrow haggle over a worm. I asked her what made her happiest during her life. Martha's thoughts spewed forth like lava from a volcano. "My husband was rough around the edges like me, but he had a kind heart. Together we made a family that was the opposite of what I had."

Without a beat, she shared about the close relationship she had with her facility roommate. I suppose a bond had been forged through similar traumas like the ones formed between bunkmates confined to a prison cell. In short order came . . . Kat and Ladybug . . . pumpkin pie with swirls of real cream . . . an icy, shandy-style beer on a muggy day . . . a Belgium Fat Tire ale with a burger smothered in fried onions with steak sauce, and the memories of miles trekked across the country with her motorcycle club.

She went back in years to recount her excitement over discovering the early Harley magazine *Hog*. Martha let out a sliver of a whistle when she described the features of her own Harley bike: chrome accents, a glossy burgundy finish, and leather saddlebags. Those comforting memories revived her spirit.

"Bullet was slick," she said.

Everyone needs a Bullet or a BB, I had thought at the time.

We traded stories and trials. Her fears? She wanted to know what would happen after she died. She had two specific concerns: Would her parents be in hell, and could I describe purgatory? I guess she had changed her mind on the existence of a Supreme Being in the afterlife. For now, I was trying to get Martha out of her head and into her heart, but we needed a break from the serious exercise of legacy-building and the possible retributions of the afterlife. Those concerns could simmer.

So, we launched into a joke-telling contest. If she won, I would have a plate of paczki, a traditional Polish dessert, delivered to her room. Her first droll attempt for our contest was truly comical. Martha, who was "mostly" Polish, announced the subject matter and then set up the joke. With a glimmer in her eye and clearing her throat, she launched into her clever thigh-slapper: "A Polish immigrant had recently arrived at a DMV in NYC and was taking an eye test to get a driver's license. The examiner showed him a large card of letters to read out loud." Martha grabbed a napkin, borrowed my pen, and scratched out these letters for me to see as she spoke: C Z A J K O W Y T Z.

Then she proceeded to the punchline. "The examiner asked: 'Can you read this?' The Polish man replied, 'Can I read it? I know that guy!'" She cackled. *She actually cackled.* I remember thinking:

Who is this woman? Watching Martha enjoy herself had been an anomaly. It was a salve for her spirit and mine. Chuckling all the way to the bakery after work, I picked up her prize of Polish dessert.

I mentioned to Martha my observations over the prior thirty minutes and then pressed "play." The upbeat attitude, the loving legacy she had been proud to articulate, the sense of gratitude, the laughter, the thoughtfulness, and the mischievousness spilled forth from the recording. Her face softened. She seemed bemused by my recording stunt. Martha searched my face and then nodded, as if to say: *Who would have thought?*

Our time had ended with a joke and a prayer. Then, I handed her a homework assignment with two questions to ponder: First, what do you think happens at the moment of death? Second, what have you learned from suffering and how did you go about rebuilding your life after you left your parents? It was a tall order. She nodded, and we agreed to meet the next morning.

At the crack of dawn, I was awake and mentally preparing for the day ahead.

Four patients were on my agenda and I was meeting with a family to enroll their father on our service late in the afternoon. When I arrived at Martha's nursing home, I set up the grill on the flagstone-lined patio on the side of the building. When I went up to get Martha, she was feeling tired, nauseous, and her cough had worsened; but she insisted we tackle the homework assignment. After checking in with the RN for a medical update, I wheeled Martha to the patio.

On the way down, I contacted our team's young RN case manager to ask about Martha's prescription for Levsin. It treated gastric emissions. Martha had colon cancer.

I settled Martha in a secluded area. The grill was lit. She said she wasn't hungry for a burger. No burgers today, but I had made good on my promise and brought a few powdery fried doughnuts with stewed plum filling in a bakery bag. I told her we were going to perform a ritual like her Indigenous ancestors had performed for the dying of their communities. She looked puzzled, and I knew she didn't feel well when she refused the paczki.

"So, you were wondering if your parents would be in hell when you got to heaven?"

She explained that after our conversations about God, it would make sense that a loving Creator might exist to chasten sinners, maintain justice, and inflict appropriate punishments, in particular. *A sentiment that a good cop could understand and endorse.*

We were making progress.

"So, you don't have to worry about them," I said. "Maybe they're learning how to love themselves and others in the next life."

I took out a pile of large index cards and asked Martha to consider devoting a card to any of these areas: forgiveness, victimization, unresolved anger, regrets, or any residual grief from the loss of her childhood innocence. Or leave them blank. She nibbled on the nub of her pencil, examined the slate-gray coals and glowing embers, and proceeded to empty her heart and mind of adolescent misery. She filled five cards. I wrote out my own set and waited.

After twenty minutes, she looked up with wet eyes. Her mind was already a simmering fire, long-kindled, that snapped and sizzled with molten bitterness. I directed her to toss the first card into the grill. Would her volatile thoughts act as an accelerant to fuel the sputtering flame into a ravenous inferno? But the fire simply shouldered the sentiments of her soul and thirst for justice like a seasoned army recruit on a special assignment.

The grill devoured each of our cards, in turn. And with them, the deepest secrets of our souls were sent flickering and swirling to the heavens. The ashy remnants of regret, sorrow, and resentment billowing skyward like the smoldering embers of incense offered at a religious service. A sense of hope taking root in the inner space that had been vacated. I explained that her Indigenous ancestors held fire ceremonies to help them stay open-minded, grounded, and kind. I could have benefitted from a *monthly* fire ceremony.

She searched her lap and shyly lifted her gaze to mine.

"Do you feel lighter? More peaceful?" I asked.

She dabbed at her eyes.

"Not quite. I owe you an apology. I'm sorry for denigrating your career."

I chuckled. "Martha, I understood; and I accept your apology."

I folded her hand in mine.

She also had another matter on her mind. "What about purgatory. Does it hurt?"

"Is that what you're most fearful of after all you've lived through?" I probed. Her entire childhood and adolescence was hell, so the concept of addressing a state of more suffering to expiate a surplus of sin before going to heaven seemed outlandish.

She asked if I was afraid of purgatory and I told her that I was not. "Purgatory is a *process* of illumination. It's liberating. Whenever I've been in a position to learn something nasty about myself, I felt disappointed in myself, deep regret, and sorrow. Shame and remorse. So, yes, it hurts. These are some of the religious issues that people want to work through before they die.

She had been baptized Roman Catholic and had grown up before the Second Vatican Council when the conception of purgatory was a fiery place of physical torment dating back to the religious and literary insights of the twelfth century. I envisioned the process of purification (purgatory) like suffering through an Enneagram class—gaining the insight and truth (self-awareness) that I hadn't obtained on earth. Not fun, but necessary.

Purification is a blessed opportunity whether on earth or after we die. It is an internal process. Think of it like the red flag coaches drop to review a sports play for accuracy. Imagine if we had an automatic and instantaneous review of our actions in real time.

God accompanies us as we look at our own bullshit. God always saw us and loved us for who we really were—our gifts, idiosyncrasies, faults, and sins. God also knew who we were meant to become. So, to experience fully the innocence, unconcealed essence of matter, and intense light that is heaven, everyone needs to see clearly and feel deeply. Just as silver and gold are refined in fire by melting them down and skimming the impurities, it makes sense that only a spiritual fire could burn away spiritual impurities.

According to Jungian analyst Donald Kalsched, "Healing our wounds is a process of *remembering* those places and experiences that have been cut off, thereby giving our disowned feelings a fully felt place in our consciousness." It didn't seem as if Martha had much of an opportunity to do that.

I asked her if she wanted me to call a priest for the Sacrament of Reconciliation. She was visibly weighing the possibility and started to speak, but then seemed to think better of it.

"Are you sure, Martha? I have some retired priests who provide the sacrament for the dying. You can reconsider it tomorrow if you're feeling better."

By the time we got back to the room, Martha was in some pain. She was scheduled to receive morphine every two hours, and yet the pain was still penetrating the opiate regimen. I didn't understand what was happening. After finally reaching our newly-hired RN, we sorted through the issue. Our supplies were low, and we were down to only six syringes. Our uncertified RN had reduced the dose to every four hours until our next shipment arrived. Did she understand that admitting to an unauthorized change in medications would place her job in jeopardy?

She assured me it was expected soon.

"How soon? In the next ten minutes?"

She reiterated that her hands were tied. Her explanation really ignited my ire.

"Procure some syringes. Borrow. Beg. Barter. Steal. I don't care; you're the RN."

I asked again about the order for Levsin, the one I had checked on hours ago. The RN said she had indeed faxed the order that morning, but when I called the pharmacy, it reported no order had been submitted. Why was the chaplain triple-checking everything? My God. This would never have happened in my first eighteen months with our company. I tried to fathom what had happened to that order.

"Did you stay to make sure the fax went through?" No, she had not. I called our office, and someone found the fax unsent, and no one had noticed.

When I started at HA in 2010, our nursing staff was stellar. Rookie mistakes such as this never happened because we didn't hire uncertified and inexperienced RNs, or if we did, they were well-trained before we turned them loose upon the dying. But experienced hospice RNs cost money.

By the time Kat and her husband walked through the door, Martha was semi-conscious and visibly uncomfortable. I sat with them and tried to address their confusion and frustration. Kat took one of her grandmother's hands, and I held the other.

I blessed Martha and recited the prayers of commendation.

I started the oxygen and left the room so Kat could spend time alone with her beloved Bacia. While I was pacing, I saw our RN administrator at the end of a long hall getting off the elevator. She carried what I assumed to be both medications. Some of our administrators had been social workers or financial managers, so this was fortunate. Just then, Kat came running out—sobbing. Martha was coughing up a lot of blood and bile. I told Kat and her husband to wait in the family lounge at the end of the hall.

When I reached the room, Martha was groaning and had the look of panic in her eyes. I raised the head of the bed, wiped Martha's bloody face, and grabbed a fresh gown. After sliding on clean gloves, I changed her clothing and then watched our administrator infuse the drugs. I wasn't on-call, but the RN, Kat, and I stayed with Martha until she died three hours later, just after ten o'clock. Five minutes before she passed, she sat up, extended her arms, and looked toward the window with a glow on her face. No one was visible to us.

"Papa i mama," she murmured. And then she laid back against the sheets.

The RN checked for a pulse. She was gone. Kat looked at me for a bit of reassurance at Martha's final, hair-raising posture. A smile broke on my face, one of relief and joy. I assured Kat that I'd seen this happen before, and then we both started to cry. It was always such a relief to get them over the threshold to the eternal.

The door that didn't reveal itself until a person was ready swung wide for Martha. The Escort had been waiting. *Ah, Rumi. The secrets that have been revealed during these last weeks.*

My gaze drifted to the "old lady" sitting on the windowsill. Her white, fuzzy, spiked hair had spawned a single pink flower. That cactus usually blooms in late winter, but it had bloomed early. A harbinger. The pincushion cactus had thrived after all, just like Martha. God had protected the sergeant for eternity—molding her, rearranging atoms, turning her around and around. In the light of darkness—God had fashioned a new creation.

The Velveteen Rabbit was one of my favorite books to read to patients. It's about what it's like to grow into one's elderly years and the cost of loving.

The Skin Horse said, "When someone loves you for a long, long time, not just to play with, but really loves you, then you become real."

"Does it hurt?" asked the Rabbit.

"Sometimes," said the Skin Horse, for he was always truthful. "When you are real, you don't mind being hurt."

I came to deeply respect Martha and my grieving for her had already begun. She refused to spiritualize, explain away, or ignore the truth of suffering in this world. Martha understood the emotional cost to work through it all. That crusty cop would've made one fine chaplain. After everything she had witnessed in her home and career, her initial protest was reasonable. She allowed the reality of her life to shake her soul. I will always remember her for that.

Seven days later, we celebrated Martha's life—all of it. The beauty, the bitterness, the sorrow, the courage, the love. I planned a small service and gave her eulogy. We commemorated her journey to become "real." In the final analysis, the Enneagram and "purgatory" are really just a purification process for becoming real.

A Company Ruse Backfired

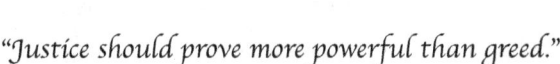

"Justice should prove more powerful than greed."
Fred Rogers, Presbyterian minister and television host

WALKING THROUGH THE DOOR AFTER WORK ON FRIDAY with Martha's last hours circling my thoughts, I found Mark in bed. He said he felt terrible and looked it. I was alarmed. His physicians were treating his staph infection with antibiotics, but these measures were not helping. So, they sent him home with a different medication. He had an appointment the next week with the cardiac-transplant team at University Hospital in Madison. For the time being, Mark was off the transplant list. Our third rebuff. I watched the light at the end of the tunnel dim with each health crisis that disqualified him, and Mark's resolve with it.

Mayo Clinic had given Mark a prognosis of two to five years to live without a transplant. We were in year three. We had never discussed abandoning the transplant option. Closing that particular door was too overwhelming and frightening. We often fell asleep at night holding hands and praying for the call that would summon us to another chance for health, wholeness, and a shot at living a decent life.

I did quietly consider hospice for Mark, but it seemed like a betrayal. Giving up. He was just fifty-nine-years-old. And his cardiac team in Madison repeatedly assured us, "We will transplant him." He was a fighter, but there were periods when he wanted to give up—it was exhausting staying viable for a premier position on a transplant list.

It's hard for nonmedical folks to believe that Mark wasn't appropriate for hospice care even with a diagnosis of end-stage heart failure. I take that back; he was appropriate. But he had grueling choices to make. His transplant regimen required him to consume thirty-six pills each day to stay alive until a heart was available. Mark clung to life with an ejection-fraction rate of 40 percent. Normal is between 55 and 70 percent. The nasty side effects from such a hefty load of drugs took a toll on the quality of his life. And mine. But not on our love.

I was preparing a tomato sauce for dinner when an email arrived from the human resources division of our corporate office in Michigan. The company's management style had become so oppressive that many of us referred to the head honchos at the corporate office in Bay City, Michigan, as "The Capitol," the seat of the brutal and totalitarian government in *The Hunger Games*. It started the day our staff manager sauntered down the corridors of our offices to remind us that a corporate executive was arriving that afternoon, and proclaimed, "Heads are going to roll." Was this Paris in the eighteenth century? Who talks like that to loyal, hard-working employees?

In the email, Susan, the human resources director, outlined the changes for my employee health care coverage. She wrote, "It would be in your *best interest, and ours,* if you could switch to a different health insurance plan. It is possible that the exact benefits you enjoy now won't be available in the new plan. Please take the weekend to think it over, but we need a response ASAP. Call me on Monday. We can go over the details."

A quick response would not be forthcoming. The request didn't even make sense. But if it really was in my "best interest" to switch, then I wasn't concerned. Mark was approved for a heart transplant and had started the protocols with our current insurance plan. We were all set. I guess we would just transfer the transplant to the new plan. I called a colleague. No, she hadn't heard about the company switching providers. Nothing was in the online company newsletter.

I didn't want to worry Mark, but I stewed about it all weekend while he slept on and off. Monday morning arrived overcast and rainy. Thunder was rolling in. A bad omen. Mark was still miserable. I got him settled, started the infusion of the new antibiotics (as they had instructed), and called a neighbor to check in on him during the day. I only had two weeks of personal days a year and we needed to save it for the transplant.

Mark used a plastic two-level tackle box as a pill sorter. Nothing else was big enough to handle thirty-six pills a day, seven days a week. The tackle box was the color of canned peas; the hue was anemic, like his complexion and level of energy, and it dominated our home and lives for three years. It seemed as if that putrid box took on a larger-than-life personality of its own, taunting us from its station in the kitchen. Reminding us that Mark's life was no longer his own.

I understood how children felt with the Elf on a Shelf monitoring their every move during the holidays. It was a dispenser of life-giving tablets and horrid side effects alike. Those finger-tip-sized pebbles of plastic were all that was keeping him above ground. That, and the hope of a heart transplant.

I locked my office door and dialed Susan. My list of questions was extensive enough to consume a twenty-foot-long scroll of parchment. I wished I had been in her office to unroll it ceremoniously, watch it gather speed across her floor, and sweep out into the hallway right up to the polished Silvano-Sassetti wingtips of our hospice owner. She answered after the third ring and launched into the plan for switching us to another provider.

"So, here's the deal. Mrs. Torinus, if you decide to switch, you will no longer receive your paycheck from Hospice Advantage. Instead, it will be issued from a company called Allen of Bay."

She rattled on, "One perk that we can't promise is dental benefits."

Dental coverage was the least of our worries, but we were accustomed to receiving regular cleanings and common procedures on our current plan.

"Susan, the only 'perk' we are desperate to retain is the heart transplant." She brushed past my comment like a streetsweeper on a deadline.

"Can you get back to me in twenty-four hours with your decision?" I pictured her perfunctorily crossing out the pesky insurance item from her long to-do list. It was business as usual in Bay City, Michigan.

The stark omission from the corporate office about the transplant hit me with the force of an unexpected tidal wave. We were in the middle of the transplant protocols, for God's sake. My head was exploding with even more questions.

Am I the only employee in my agency switching to a different provider? What about the employees in Alabama and the other twelve states? How is it in my "best interest" to accommodate this request? What is Allen of Bay? Could the transplant still proceed with a different insurance provider? Wasn't this the company of "compassion"? Why would it be in the company's "best interest" to switch me off our current health insurance? That made no sense. I was *so* naïve.

I tried to ask those pertinent questions, but Susan stonewalled me. Did they think that Mark and I had just fallen off a turnip truck? But she had no clue who she was up against; I've never been a shrinking violet. I was steaming when I dialed the number for the new health insurance provider in Iowa. But I reminded myself that the receptionist who would answer was only the messenger and most likely sat in a stuffy cubicle, doing her best to help prospective clients. After she transferred me to an agent, it didn't take long to reach the crux of the matter for clients with pre-existing conditions.

After the agent and I had dispensed with the usual pleasantries, she cautioned me. "No, Maryclaire, your husband would not be a candidate for a heart transplant if he switched policies. I would never recommend that." *Of course not. No one with an ounce of compassion or a working brain would recommend that.*

It was clear my company got the same feedback from the agent before it pitched the swap to me. "The Capitol" understood the dire ramifications we faced without a transplant—Mark would die. *Or at least, he would die way before they said he was supposed to die.* Make no mistake about it, our hospice advertisement and promise to provide "Care, Comfort, and Offer Compassion" did not extend to employees or their family members.

I was trembling when I hung up. I Googled "Allen of Bay." It was located in Miami, Florida, owned by HA, and had one employee listed. What type of subsidiary had only one employee? Apparently, my naivety had no bounds. I noticed that the company management listed on the website included many of the same people involved with our company.

My next call was to an attorney who specialized in health-insurance fraud. I wasn't sure what was actually occurring here, but I needed professional advice. I didn't have the time, energy, or money to push back on what seemed like an unethical scheme at minimum, but this was a life-or-death situation.

My attorney suggested we send a cease-and-desist letter; a toe-testing maneuver. But I wasn't in the mood for "toe-testing;" we didn't have time for that. A dive into the deep end is what I had lobbied for. We sent the letter. It was a relief to have an expert on my side because Mark had no idea what was afoot.

I waited. And waited. And waited.

I wasn't sure what my next steps would be if they ignored the letter or called our bluff. Lacking the money to press them with a lawsuit, I did what I knew how to do best—I prayed. Between my intense work with the dying, Mark's terminal condition, and the antics of my company, I felt overwhelmed. Exhausted. And frightened.

I asked my attorney why our company would do this. He speculated that if our hospice company was owned by a private equity firm, the debt load that they forced the company to bear added pressure to reduce overhead. If HA was self-insuring to reduce health insurance costs, they would have an incentive to offload employees whose families consumed a lot of expensive health care to a cheaper plan with less coverage. He also surmised that I wasn't the only HA employee in their network across the country being intimidated to switch to a cheaper plan.

And what about the "Allen of Bay" reference? I inquired. His theory at the time was that it was nothing more than a "shell" company—a legal entity that has no purpose other than to be an instantaneous pass-through of funds to provide insulation from liability. In other words, it was illegal to pick and choose who stays on a health insurance plan.

I didn't understand. Wouldn't the infusion of millions of dollars into our company boost our resources and staffing? The end result would've been excellent patient care and happy employees. But quite often, the opposite was true.

Ten days later, I received a terse call from Susan retracting the proposal for switching our health insurance. No explanation. No apology. No hand-wringing. No shame-filled stuttering. Our "toe-testing" maneuver must have been enough to roil the corporate waters. I fantasized about what was really going through her head during our call: *Well, we gave it our best shot, but I guess you didn't just fall off the turnip truck. No harm, no foul. Thanks for playing.* And then she would have swiped her hands back and forth with a swishing sound as if to shake loose the leftover crumbs from a failed baking experiment.

Doctors are not the only professionals who should take the Hippocratic Oath. Anyone involved in health care—all owners, executives, managers, and investors—should also promise that they will uphold ethical standards within their businesses for top-notch patient care. Medical care demands that patients should always be the primary stakeholders.

My attorney had surmised that the company would drop the nasty ruse. I did understand that transplants were expensive; the cost could be as high as a million dollars. But didn't insurance companies hire backup companies for expensive medical procedures?

HA washed their hands of their foray into criminal activity because I blew the whistle on them. Well, sort of. I don't believe it's whistleblowing if the shrill sounds of protest only ricochet within the walls of the offending company. After I had calmed down, I emailed Susan with a demand to reimburse my legal fees. It was a bold request, and I had a lot to lose . . . like our livelihood. But between these insurance shenanigans and the increased negligence in patient care occurring, I needed to act. And I prayed. Big time.

Without my lawyers knowledge, I affixed a minor threat to my urgent request: I would report this foray into unethical behavior to the state of Wisconsin and to CMS.

A week later, an $800 dollar check arrived from the corporate office in Bay City, Michigan. Afterward, I explained the sordid details to Mark. The incompetence, swagger, and carelessness of my company shocked him. To my benefit, they had left an unintended paper trail of documents in their wake. The stress of remaining with this company was mounting. What was their endgame?

I felt as if I was losing my soul and I wasn't even dying.

The Quantum Leap

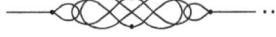

"The eyes of a person who is dying are the clearest mirrors I have ever known. In their gaze, there is simply no place to hide."
Frank Ostaseski, Buddhist teacher and founding director of the Zen Hospice Project

THE AMBULANCE RACED TO THE NEAREST HOSPITAL, TWENty-five minutes away, with sirens blaring and lights flashing. My daughter and I were in my Subaru Crosstrek, directly behind it. But the paramedics warned us not to match their pace. The driver accelerated and the traffic in their cross hairs slowed to a standstill as the vehicle streaked by.

There was no room for me at Mark's side with the crush of lifesaving equipment and the business of resuscitation going on. So, while the emergency medical technicians sped toward more sophisticated emergency room equipment and battled my husband's thready pulse, my daughter and I pumped the brakes at red lights, yellow lights, and stop signs. What progress we had managed was soon impeded by the rush-hour traffic. I pounded the steering wheel and blared the horn at the drivers paused at green lights, heads down, immersed in their texts and emails. With every passing mile, my husband's final minutes were dispersed like the exhaust streaming from the tailpipe stalled in front of us. It didn't take long before we could no longer hear sirens.

By the time we got to the ER, he was gone.

Mark died on a Monday. Around the dinner hour. August 21, 2013. My daughter Anne, twenty-nine years old, uttered an otherworldly moan when a doctor delivered the news, and I gathered her into my arms. She wanted to go home with a friend, and I let her. This was the time for me to say goodbye to her father. A nurse took my arm and guided me toward one of the emergency rooms—a huge room with every piece of life-saving equipment a tattered body would ever need. But it wasn't enough to save my beloved Mark.

My husband was lying on a gurney in the center of the vast room still attached to the intubation equipment. The overhead lighting was garish, and the brilliant reflection of it off the sterile-looking steel hit hard. The room felt cold and forbidding. Mark looked so alone. I rushed to him.

The paramedics had been aggressive in their attempts to save him, a man who was barely sixty and on a transplant list. When they arrived at our home, Mark was lying on our bed and I was on top of him, desperately attempting CPR. A hard surface would've been better, but I didn't want to roll him off the bed. We had high mattresses, and even our sixty-seven-pound Labrador needed a ramp to get up and down. As they worked on Mark, I heard a crunching sound. No one stopped. No one looked up. His ribs had fractured. Tears rolled down my cheeks.

A medic tossed medical supplies toward me to open. I floundered and finally tore an opening with my teeth. Every second counted. It was all hands on deck. Mark would have hated those extreme measures on his behalf, but we had not gotten far enough in our end-of-life discussions to consider a "do not resuscitate" order. But he was still young and the chance of obtaining a viable heart wasn't something to pass up. Besides, I was not ready to let him die. And on and on it went.

So, in a moment of panic I lost my resolve: the promise to relieve him of three long years of suffering if it came to that. In hindsight,

I believe his condition had indeed come to a crossroads that night. But the stakes were high, and I couldn't afford to make mistakes in judgment. I needed to err on the side of hope. It happened so quickly.

I had driven Mark to University Hospital in Madison about a week earlier because he was having trouble breathing. He dubbed me "Mario," after the race car driver Mario Andretti, as I sped the fifty miles to their campus. I'd called ahead so the cardiac department would be ready for us. Where were the officers when speeding was absolutely necessary and deadly appropriate?

I stayed with Mark at the hospital for the following weekend and returned to work that Monday morning. His older brother Tom offered to drive him home later that afternoon. The cardiologists called to tell me that he was stable enough to be discharged.

Tom dropped him off, and we chatted for a bit. Then Mark and I were left sitting in the sunroom. He asked me to move closer and hold his hand. I scraped a chair across the floor and wedged it between his lounger and the sofa. Our knees were touching. Deep down, I think we both knew what was about to happen and denial settled in. Sometimes I had trouble facing the hard truth of things.

He rubbed his arm and said streaks of pain were pulsating up and down. I knew what that type of arm pain meant in his condition. He must have sensed something wasn't right. And me? I had done everything wrong after he walked through our front door that Monday. I puttered, checked email, and fed the dog, never thinking that day would be *the day*. *The Day for Dying.* They had sent him home, after all. It started out like any other day in a long line of days living with end-stage heart failure. We barely kissed because damn it, no one told us he was going to die that night, within two hours.

And then I remembered the card that fell out of my book that day on the lake: "At the end of my life, I want your hand in mine, and then I will join the stars and orbit around you forever."

Fear froze time in that instant. I felt as if I would slug through molasses for the rest of my life. Less than three minutes after he reached for my hand, I guided him to our bed. He wasn't settled for more than a minute when his eyes rolled back. He didn't cry out. I gasped at the stark-white bulging sclera of his eyes and fumbled to punch 911. Frightened, I launched into my version of cardiac resuscitation. It had been a while since I was trained in it.

Do I compress or breathe first? How many do I do? For God's sake, Maryclaire, it doesn't matter. Just do something. Anything.

I remembered to place the heels of my hands in the middle of his chest and pushed down as hard as I could. And then two forceful breaths, more compressions . . . but suddenly, I couldn't remember how many I'd done. I started crying. "This is not the time for tears," I chastised myself. "Get a hold of yourself. Breathe for him." Mark looked no better. Maya hid under the bed.

For a moment, it seemed a blessing to cover his mouth with my own. Those lips were comforting and familiar amid the utter chaos. The sweetness of his breath surprised me, but then I realized his system was shutting down. His breath smelled like nail polish remover. Why did I always have to think like a chaplain? Why did I have to know so freaking much about dying and death? *God, please help me.*

That night, at the hospital, I asked if I could spend time with Mark. Alone. Thankfully, it was a slow night in the emergency department and they didn't need the room. That was a parachute of grace from God. A shield for my heart. An RN positioned a gurney alongside Mark, and I climbed up. I planted kisses on his pale cheek, placed my arm across his motionless chest, and whimpered my love and regrets into his ear. My tears dampened the sleeve of his flannel shirt. This wasn't how it was supposed to be. I'd rather be anyone else right now.

My love language after his debilitating heart attack had been to work my tail off to keep our health insurance and pay our bills. I know he appreciated my role, but I still felt guilty for being more available to my patients than to him at times.

I would have laid next to him all night had they allowed it. But a hospital was a place for the recovering and the rescued.

Time passed on that metal gurney between suffocating cascades of grief and poignant memories. Watching him waving those slimy fish trophies toward me that day on the lake. His mischievous grin flashed before me. *My love.* His hand felt cold beneath mine. I slipped his wedding ring onto my finger, next to my own.

If Mark had been looking down at me from the stars, as he had promised, he would have seen me clinging to his corpse and sobbing. I knew every inch of that lifeless body—inside and out. We lay there like two star-crossed lovers. One dead, and one wishing she was. He had been my life partner for thirty-eight years of marriage and some change. And my good friend since fifth grade. Now, he was gone. Gone in an instant. Poof. Just like that. I was now a widow. Alone.

Mark must have felt tremendous relief to rid himself of that old husk of a body and all of its aches and pain. He had been so weary of the unending physical decline as he waited for the transplant: Driving to an errand and getting lost, frequent falls, and needing a change of clean clothes at hand. As he phrased it, "I shit my pants again." Downing dozens of pills each day wreaks havoc on bodily functions.

Good riddance, he must've exclaimed, like a woman wrestling her girdle, bra, and hosiery to the bedroom floor at the end of a demanding workday. Ah, such liberation.

It would have been enough for me if the transplant had given Mark more time, regardless of his post-surgery condition, but he told me that he didn't want to keep living if he couldn't fly fish, hunt, or do what he loved most. And then he told me over dinner one night that he was certain he would die before me and he felt relief. Mark assured me that I would be okay without him, but he couldn't live without me. I never asked why. It didn't matter. Our dinner conversations had definitely become more gut-wrenching as his heart failed to cling to life.

But I wouldn't be okay without him. I would miss meeting him after work at a pub for a beer and a burger to catch up on the day.

I would miss our last minute excursions to drive nowhere and everywhere just to explore and watch sunsets. I would miss our pillow talks in bed, probing his thoughts and ideas.

On the other hand, I knew I could eventually live a good life without him, but I'd always be aware that something was not quite right. He was my soul mate, so I could never be fully satisfied without him. I would have to fully depend on God. *Said the chaplain.*

The staff approached our gurneys and informed me that the medical team responsible for harvesting tissue had arrived and they needed to move Mark to the hospital morgue. He had always wanted to donate his organs to help others if it came to that. I laid my hand over his motionless chest and told him that I would have accepted his engagement ring all over again. In a heartbeat.

As I walked from the room, my thoughts flashed back to the recent weekend when he was in the hospital. Mark was unusually relaxed. We laughed and joked about silly things. He was calm and carefree; he teased and flirted. More than anything else, he radiated serenity. We hadn't been this light-hearted together in a long while. He even looked younger and bright-eyed—like old times, before the assault on his health rearranged our lives to the realities of before and after his heart attack.

It was such a remarkable change that I felt a renewed sense of hope and mentioned it to Mark. The serenity permeated the entire room and it seemed to encircle his head and face with a glow, as if an extension of his mood. It was so noticeable.

Recently, I read a book by Allan J. Hamilton, MD, called *The Scalpel and The Soul.* He was a Harvard-educated neurosurgeon who wrote about a sphere of light that appeared to surround many of his patients' faces shortly before they died. An inexplicable warning? Mark died exactly twenty-four hours after I noticed the light. I'd never witnessed that glow in a hospice patient, although on their deathbeds, a few patients told me they'd seen hazy images of family members, angels, or Jesus at the foot of their beds.

My explanation for the phenomenon was that perhaps Mark's soul was already preparing to leave this world. I researched and found extensive medical literature that described energy-field changes that occurred during the death transition.

A friend drove me home from the hospital. As I watched neighborhood after neighborhood pass by, I pondered all I would miss about Mark. The list was long. As I prepared for bed that night, my arms ached for his embrace. Sleep arrived slowly. Our king-sized bed, no longer a comforting rendezvous for our nightly pillow talks, felt the size of Noah's Ark with one passenger. I looked over to his side where he had laid just a few hours earlier, grabbed his pillow in my arms, and cried myself to sleep.

Some nights, I turned his CPAP machine on and let the cool air waft over me and pretended he was still lying there. Who would rub my back, zip up my dress, and take me dancing? Who would witness my life now?

Mark had wanted to donate his organs after he died, but the medical team found them in poor condition. His ailing heart could not pump enough blood for the last three years to keep his organs viable enough to transplant. That discovery made me cry. He must have felt so terrible waiting for that second chance at life, but hardly ever complained.

However, they were able to harvest those beautiful brown eyes for their corneas and other needed tissue. A few months later, I received a letter from the Lions Eye Bank of Wisconsin informing me that a woman in Two Rivers could now see because of Mark's generosity.

It's not possible to transplant the iris, or I would have combed the streets of that small town searching for the eyes that captured my friendship, my heart, and my life. Still, Mark granted another human being the chance to see what she could only imagine before.

The fourth-century theologian and mystic Gregory of Nyssa believed that "within each human soul there existed a divine element, a kind of 'inner eye' capable of glimpsing something of God." So, when I die, it will be easy to find Mark without those captivating brown eyes. I'll just look for the "inner eye" of his soul.

Upon Mark's arrival at the pearly gates, I hoped St. Peter would offer him a Korbel brandy Manhattan on the rocks with mushrooms.

Mark would have relished an authentic Irish wake, but our celebration of his life was a bit more somber. However, friends regaled us with plenty of his jokes, hilarious stories, and his penchant for mischief. Apparently, at the office, Mark once said, "Don't forget to live large, die young, and leave a good-looking corpse." *My love.* Unfortunately, that was exactly what he did. He did look better in his casket than the entire last year of his life. It's amazing what make-up can accomplish.

The card that fell out of my book that day on the lake is still taped to my bedroom mirror. It gives me solace to know that Mark will orbit around me forever.

Morphine, Myths, and George

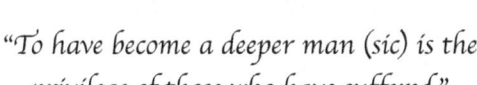

> *"To have become a deeper man (sic) is the privilege of those who have suffered."*
>
> Oscar Wilde, Irish author and playwright

After Mark's funeral, I went back to work. I had utilized all of my accumulated vacation days, but a colleague had extracted three extra days for me from management. I would've benefited from three months off. I wasn't ready to return to my end-of-life ministry while still grieving Mark so profoundly, but I needed the paycheck until I could navigate probate and untangle the life insurance issues. I felt as if I had been run over by a cement truck; I was emotionally drained. But life goes on, right? And bills need to be paid.

Thankfully, the new patient allocated to me on my hasty return was a delightful middle-aged man with a witty, self-depracating humor. George was a middle-school social science teacher. He was a widower with two daughters. His stay on our service was uneventful until his last night on earth. George's pain was increasing as he approached the active stage of dying. That stage is similar to the last part of labor—often referred to as *the transition*—and as mothers know, it is intense and painful.

When I left him at five o'clock, he was tucked in and comfortable. I called our second-shift RN who would contact our medical director to order stronger pain medication, if needed, and other antidotes for symptom control. It would be delivered immediately. George would be comfortable throughout the night, and our third-shift RN would check in on him.

I contacted George's children who had planned to stay with him for the evening and I also delivered an update to our on-call chaplain who would visit. Our RN received confirmation from the pharmacy that the medications had arrived. The nursing home CNA would deliver the prescriptions when she passed medications on the second shift. I left for the day confident that he was in good hands.

The next morning, I received the news that George had died around dawn. As planned, our third-shift RN had him on her rotation and she found the middle-school social science teacher in intense pain when she arrived in the middle of the night. She discovered that his subsequent doses of morphine were not documented and no medications were locked in the cabinet in his room. I tried to imagine the scene as she confronted the medication passer.

Surprisingly, the nursing home CNA admitted that she had only thrown out the stronger medication—the morphine—which had severely affected George's level of pain for the remaining hours of his life. Our RN repeated to our staff how the facility aide had explained to her (in a self-righteous tone) that morphine can kill a patient and it was her duty to intervene when necessary. She said it was her moral responsibility to act on his behalf. We were shocked.

I came to understand through the years that sometimes hospice care is only as competent as the nursing home it contracts with. George was a prime example. Our RNs tried to educate nursing home employees on hospice care. After all, nursing homes are still considered the primary care givers of patients in hospice.

Often, the salaries of those medication passers were lower than minimum wage, and many took on double shifts to make ends meet, so a revolving door filled with nursing assistants was typical everywhere. Consequently, trying to train nursing home employees about the specifics of professional pain management in hospice care seemed a never-ending task.

We learned at the next medical meeting that our company did not complain to the administration of that facility or to the State Division of Quality Assurance. We had a lot of patients at that facility, and apparently, we didn't want to jeopardize our hospice contract with them. The medical directors believed it irresponsible to apprise George's family of the awful turn of events for his last six hours because it was a matter of water over the dam. There would be no justice for George. We kept it completely under wraps.

Our company didn't provide ongoing education for our clinical staff while I worked there, but our hospice RNs and physicians assured our interdisciplinary teams that morphine prescribed to control symptoms and pain at the end of life had a minimal risk of hastening death. In their experience, when prescribed appropriately, the risk of respiration depression was vastly overestimated. And it's important to understand that not everyone needs opioids in their last hours; its utilization depends on many factors. Ultimately, it comes down to trusting your hospice team.

However, I did encounter family members that worried about the effects of morphine on hastening death. It seemed that the underlying concern for some religious families had to do with the spiritual benefit of willfully accepting suffering as Christ had. To me, the torture and killing of Jesus was evil.

Unrelenting pain and severe suffering that is not addressed is immoral, which is why we euthanize our beloved pets when we can't ease their pain or extend their lives. Indeed, some suffering is a part of living, and we can use our own suffering to nurture empathy and compassion for others who are undergoing adversity and misery. But the carefully administered use of opioids for hospice patients for control of moderate to severe pain and dyspnea is ethical. Incidentally, receiving morphine to ease breathing and provide severe pain relief is part of the natural dying process.

Personally, my take on the issue of pain management is that I want my pain addressed at the end, and if I die ten hours sooner, it's worth the tradeoff.

That sad episode for George occurred when Sentinel Capital Partners still owned HA. It was autumn of 2013. Their firm had been plumping up our image for a subsequent sale. Losing a contract and a lot of patients because of the ignorance of a nursing home CNA would not be in their best interests. In fact, in October 2015, the NYC equity firm did announce on their website that "having achieved their *investment objectives* with HA, it had sold to strategic buyer, Compassus Hospice."

It was also advertised on that same site that "since Sentinel's original investment, HA grew organically and through acquisitions, with operations in more than 60 locations in 14 states throughout the Midwest, Southeast, and South." This was never about pumping money into stellar patient care; it was always about wealth generation. The scales were lopsided. And like so many others, George got caught in the economic crossfire.

On my way home from work, I could not lose sight of how our company chose to handle that frightening incident. That entire episode intensified my loneliness. I missed Mark. Normally, what happened to George would've been on the top of my agenda for our pillow talk at the end of a long day. Our company continued to make compromises with our patients. I couldn't stand on the sidelines any longer pretending to be deaf and dumb. I could hear Mark's voice in my head.

Stop being shocked, and do something. You know what to do. You're going to have to leave. The sooner the better.

But how would I manage the finances? I'm tired. Starting over somewhere else is not an option.

You will be fine. You have my life insurance policy and Social Security. And you can always go back to your beloved teaching career. I will be with you.

Easy for you to say, you're not here to help me.

I felt so overwhelmed. Still working full time, I'd also navigated my way through probate and then I untangled our assets vaulted in an international bank during my noon hours. Those complicated negotiations led me into a judge's chamber. I won. I disliked corporate banking as much as I detested ticking timepieces. My biggest pet peeve? Passwords. Code phrases that dominated life like our pea-green pill sorter had. Pins to open up, close down, enter in, access, authenticate, reveal, protect, and maneuver through. Life had gotten so complicated and stressful. And that only applies to the small, insignificant stuff.

I yearned for Door County, the Bay, and the gulls buoyant on a robust breeze.

I understood now why Mark wanted to die before me. Sometimes, just getting up and dressed every day was too much for him. Procuring a new mortgage in our situation was nearly unachievable. Inspite of solid credit, banks don't look kindly on a man who had suffered a massive heart attack and was left unable to work full-time. We had just sold our lovely retirement home but with Mark's three-year prognosis and my one year of hospice work under my belt, they didn't want to gamble on us. Every week, for months, Wells Fargo Bank pestered us for more and more financial documentation. All we had left to offer was our first-born son. Dad, this wasn't fair.

A Gold Mine

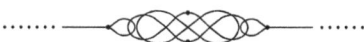

"Read, learn, work it up, go to the literature. Information is control."
Joan Didion, *The Year of Magical Thinking*

After five years with Hospice Advantage, I left the company in 2014. The number of patients had dribbled down to about fifty from a number almost triple that when I started. The administration was shedding the staff that hadn't already been nudged aside or fired.

The policy going forward was to keep employees who had seniority. I did not, but the company offered me a per diem chaplain position to help with on-call hours for the second and third shifts. The corporate office had to offer a bone to the woman who had been awarded the *National Heart of Compassion Award* given annually by the families of patients.

It took me only three seconds to weigh the merits of staying or leaving. I couldn't get my desk emptied fast enough. By the spring of 2014, my respect for this company had dwindled to almost nothing, just like our patient census and staffing quotas.

I hadn't planned on drafting a book about my experiences when I hauled my crate of supplies to the car, but I was curious about why our company took such a nosedive from its original mission and brand. None of my colleagues had a clue, and upper management and the new medical director who might know weren't free to discuss it.

So, I trudged to a local bookstore chain and immersed myself in the banality of staring at a computer screen for hours as I pored over hundreds and hundreds of hospice titles: *Nursing for Hospice Care*, *Palliative Radiation for Cancer Patients in Hospice*, and *Effective Pain Management in Hospice*. I wasn't sure what I was searching for, but a title eventually popped up that seemed a contender: *Changing the Way We Die*. The copyright date was 2013, the period in which I was interested.

The premise of that book, by award-winning journalists Sheila Himmel and Fran Smith, was that the quality of end-of-life care within the hospice movement had been declining for a decade. Like a police dog sniffing for drugs, it seemed as if I was on a viable trail. Emboldened, I bought the book.

When I glanced at the table of contents, nothing caught my attention until chapter seven, *"Inside the Catch-22 of Hospice."* A provocative title. The authors discussed the confusing Medicare rules for hospice care, the burden on caregivers who chose hospice at home, and how the hidden difficulties in some sectors of hospice care could prevent a good dying experience. My God, wasn't dying difficult enough without adding the confusion of last-minute mistakes by hospice providers?

I continued to flip through the rest of the chapters and didn't stop until chapter twelve, *"Dying for Dollars."* This chapter opened my eyes with its wealth of golden nuggets about the business side of hospice. Hundreds of companies were making fortunes caring for dying people. Who knew?

The growth of the for-profit, corporate hospice enterprise outlined in chapter twelve started in 1989 when Medicare began funding hospice services. Was the decline in service unique to our company, or a widespread problem in the hospice industry?

The narrative didn't hit the bull's eye I was hoping for until the first two sentences of paragraph eight in chapter twelve: "A typical financial newcomer to the hospice space in 2008 was Sentinel Capital Partners (SCP), a Manhattan-based equity firm with a mission *to generate attractive investment returns for lower, middle-market companies.*"

On December 14, 2012, it was SCP that bought Hospice Advantage, our chain with fifty-six providers across the Midwest and South, which they added to a diverse portfolio of companies including Huddle House family restaurants; Trussbilt LLC, a manufacturer of steel doors for prisons; Spinrite, a yarn maker; and National Spine & Pain Centers.

There it was in black and white.

So, professional investors bought our company. I went back through the notes in my patient files starting in late 2011. It was during that period that our clinicians were witnessing the decline in patient care and resources, and the noticeable change in the company culture.

Paydirt.

That revelation was the gold mine that I had never expected to find. The truth that would take me down a path I didn't intend on taking. It startled me. Yet, I was relieved to have stumbled upon a motivation for the drastic change in the company mission. All of the hasty employee departures, sparse resources, and rush to increase admissions began to make sense. I wasn't imagining anything. I wasn't an instigator or a perfectionist. Histrionics was not my thing. This was real.

That day, my questions were satisfied and months of conjecture about the change in our policies shifted to credible assumptions. Now what? Mark would've known exactly what to do with the recovery of this new data. I heard his voice once again in my head: *Now that you've come up against the truth, sit your butt in a chair, and get to work. Write.*

Finding that particular hospice book was not circumstantial; it was waiting for me. I was meant to find it. What had once appeared vague and reeked of confusion now leapt out at me from a publication based on sound journalism.

My heart was pumping. It all crystalized. The private-equity owners of our hospice valued profits over the comfort of patients. They valued profit over staff safety and training. They valued profit over the health and lives of the families of employees. Immediately, I looked up Sentinel Capital Partners and locked onto their website: "Sentinel's mission is to generate attractive investment returns by providing private equity to talented executives and then helping them build great businesses and *to realize their boldest dreams.*

What were the boldest dreams of the president of Hospice Advantage and his top management team?

The website had outlined the goals of private equity in hospice care: Acquire companies with borrowed money, recapitalize the structure, strip the assets, and cut staff while increasing the product (more patients). This process seemed similar to the reality TV shows such as: *Love It or List It, Flip or Flop,* and *Million Dollar Listing.* Likewise, the private-equity (PE) method of making money is to purchase companies that have value and can be improved. They enhance its marketability through a rapid undertaking of development, streamline their operations to increase the revenue, and sell the finished product. Unlike the reality TV shows who clean up the site, remove the construction tools, and stage the updated homes with lavish furnishings; end-of-life investors often leave suffering patients, distraught families, and disgruntled staff in their wake. Our interdisciplinary teams were forced to deal with the harm to patients and the adverse side effects of the financial process.

I don't have a problem with private equity or venture capitalists per se; I am a venture capitalist. I invest in an international company that produces carbon negative materials, and in hybrid chick-pea seed production. But I don't invest dollars in the dying.

Robert Ciardi, the managing partner of Provident Healthcare Partners oversaw the public investment-banking service for privately held companies and described his company's role with HA: "Our relationship with Hospice Advantage dates back to 2012, when we represented the organization through a financial reorganization and ultimate recapitalization with SCP." Ciardi verified SCP's goals for our company.

He added, "We were thrilled at the success that HA has had over the last three years under the guidance and stewardship with SCP and its sale to Compassus Hospice. HA is recognized for their mission of providing superior care to end-of-life patients."

I realized his public statement for what it was—a slick fabrication of the truth for a positive public endorsement and image management. It was all hype.

I never considered my hospice patients as products in a business portfolio or as financial assets comparable to restaurant chains, industrial spools of yarn, or steel door manufacturers. From what I've read, a product in a diverse portfolio must meet a company's financial objectives. So, SCP bought our hospice operations to grow the company and then sold it to Towerbrook Capital Partners, owners of Compassus Hospice, in 2015. It's nearly impossible to keep track of all of the mergers and acquisitions our company went through before the security chains were wound through the door handles at our hospice entrance in Pewaukee.

I finally had an inkling of what happened on the financial side of the company while we, the clinical staff, were working to fulfill our original mission advertised on area billboards: "Care, Comfort, and Compassion for the Entire Family." In the months leading up to the sale of our company to SCP, the mission of HA had surreptitiously changed. Our owner hired SCP to boost profit margins. Often, owners stay on as consultants after a sale. I noticed that the company stationery had started to list our former boss as the president, instead of the owner but I'd thought nothing of it.

The new vision? A singular bottom line. The new bottom line? To make a substantial profit on the backs of the dying. I thought it ironic that our new owner's firm was named *Sentinel* Capital Partners. What is a sentinel? A guard, one who stands in place to keep watch over something. To protect it.

But these *sentinels* were not hired to keep watch and protect our dying patients; their priority was to safeguard the investments of the purchasing agents—their own firm, the Norwood Mezzanine Venture Capitalists (NMV) from Minneapolis, and Wells Fargo Bank who eventually purchased NMV Capitalists.

My propensity for justice and transparency made my blood boil as I read about the corporate world's feverish quest to increase their salaries and benefits into the millions and skimp on employee compensation and patient resources in hospice and in the senior care industry. I thought about John, Martha, Helen, George, and all the others who didn't receive timely palliative care, the more costly equipment, and a host of other services that were legal entitlements.

I thought about all of our employees who had to seek legal counsel for legitimate insurance plans and compensation for work-related injuries. Venturing into the business side of hospice was not my intention or plan. I was an innocent bystander, just trying to minister to my patients to the best of my ability. Prodded by the injustice of it all, I stumbled onto the right book at the right time to unravel the mystery of our company's clinical decline. I guess you could call it divine intervention.

It's confusing, but the merger and acquisition of hospices is a current business model in many large corporations. It's becoming quite clear to those of us in the hospice sector of medical care that the private equity industry and other investors are positioning to take advantage of the "boomer tsunami" in the US by investing in the home health and hospice market.

I felt destined to work at Hospice Advantage during that period. Those pearls of wisdom and excellent journalism I discovered in

Changing the Way We Die became the seeds for this book. What were the chances I would happen upon a rather obscure hospice narrative on a dusty bookstore shelf that revealed the evidence I needed to corroborate what I witnessed inside my own agency? What were the chances that the research buried in chapter twelve, paragraph eight, sentence one would catapult a chaplain into writing about the business side of dying?

There had been no evidence of the correlation between corporate greed and diminished care in the hospice industry. Until now. Until my account. I've learned that digging deep or plunging into chaos can expose the truth and help save lives. It seemed incumbent upon me to search for the truth.

After 2012, we noticed an oppressive culture seep into our offices and increased visits from the corporate office in Michigan. Everything took on an urgency that didn't synchronize with a pastoral environment for the dying. We felt the acceleration of obtrusive oversight of our work. One day, the corporate office gathered the entire staff and administered a detailed survey about office protocols, clinical practice, and staff morale.

In speaking to my colleagues, most of our collective responses to the evaluation emphasized our slide in care and our extreme frustration. Upper management was less than pleased with our first attempt and ordered a do-over. Managers suggested we employ a more "positive outlook" the second time around and also requested that we endorse our evaluations with our specific jobs within the company. At the time, we didn't understand that a glowing survey was vital to their mission to sell the company.

That survey was never about listening to us and a sincere attempt at improving our care for patients. Headquarters didn't care if their single-minded decisions impacted patients, families, and staff in a negative manner. There were bigger fish to fry. We were never the true stakeholders—the owners and investors were. Was this a case of capitalism gone awry, or business as usual? Our candid feedback was deemed harmful for their purposes and regarded with disdain. And worse? We feared retribution.

They never shared the results.

So much of my work as a chaplain revolved around spiritual consciousness—my own and that of my patients. Self-awareness is necessary for human growth and development. Therefore, a good hospice company must be managed by people who are conscious. In any sphere of life, uplifting society comes down to virtuous conduct in business, relationships, and all institutions.

The takeover of hospice companies by equity firms, venture capitalists, and banks was to expedite growth in each company for a stake in its profits. How did "growth" occur in a company where human beings were the equity or product? I reviewed my hospice journal again from 2012 to 2014, when the slide in care occurred.

Suddenly, the covert mission of our company became obvious. It explained the aggressive competitions to drastically increase our census that placed pressure on our sales team to accept patients who weren't necessarily within the six-month window of dying. I had learned from our more seasoned staff that HA had a reputation in the industry for "bending rules" to increase and maintain a high patient census.

Bloomberg writer John Authers, in his 2020 newsletter said, "Private equity-backed US companies numbered approximately 4,000 in 2006, but by 2018, that figure had doubled to about 8,000." One-quarter of those companies owned hospices. Dying has become a component of big business. To be clear, there is private equity investment and then there is *predatory* private equity. There are venture capitalists, and then there are *vulture* capitalists.

I viewed hospice chaplaincy as my life's work, but huge for-profit corporations seemed to eye hospices strictly for short-term financial gains. Investors were looking at the silver tsunami of aging baby boomers, like me, and wanted their cut. Unfortunately, the taxpayers were the ones truly paying the tab for the hospice corporations who engaged in these get-rich-quick schemes through Medicare and Medicaid.

Let Them Eat Cake

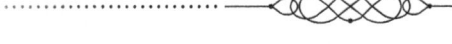

*"The first responsibility of a leader is to define reality. The last
is to say thank you. In between, the leader is a servant."*

Max De Pree, businessman and author

AFTER I HAD COME UPON THE FACTS OF HOW AN INVESTMENT firm takes over a hospice company, I checked LinkedIn to see what new enterprise our former employer was involved in. I surmised that after he sold our company to Sentinel Capital Partners in 2012, and proceeded to consult on the next sale to another private equity firm that resulted in the merger of HA with Compassus Hospice in 2015, that he might've ditched the business of hospice care. He did. In the wake of that merger, the doors of our former agency in Waukesha County had been manacled for good.

I've acknowledged that idle curiosity holds risks and creates moral mandates for prying people like me, but consumers benefit from the sacrifices, intellectual inquisitiveness, and investigative research from do-gooders, journalists, writers, social activists, and even hospice chaplains.

One of the most quoted phrases from the French Revolution is attributed to Queen Marie Antoinette, *So let them eat cake*. The peasantry of the nation were experiencing a shortage of bread, and what bread there was cost much more than they could afford. The pithy expression highlighted how deeply disconnected the wealthy rulers of France were from the peasants.

You might wonder why I inserted a popular phrase from the late eighteenth century into this memoir. First, because I had received a timely book-club selection on Marie Antoinette, and it got me thinking about more than guillotines. Second, there is a correlation between the arrogant and greedy corporations of our time and eighteenth-century royalty—both exploited the vulnerable.

And finally, I refused to capitulate to those executives and investors in our hospice company who conducted a feverish march toward fortune and pleasure on the backs of our dying patients, their families, and employees. People who, from their lofty corporate perches and catbird seats in Michigan, also seemed to scoff at lower-level employees and patients by hosting lavish corporate parties. Our hospice physicians and upper-level managers returned from Miami, Florida, with intriguing stories about the gourmet food, expensive wine, lovely hostesses, pricey entertainment, and gossip about a newly-purchased property in France.

I borrowed the phrase "let them eat cake" because the wealthy owners, senior-level managers, and investors of our hospice company were just as disconnected from the day-to-day realities of our dying patients and the issues of our employees and their families, as the French rulers were from the peasantry in the late 1700s.

In 2012, preoccupation with the recapitalization of our company rendered the owners tone deaf to our concerns and responsibilities, and they continued to remain out of touch.

So, imagine my surprise when I Googled our former owner in 2016, and the purchase of an estate fit for a king popped up on my screen. Their "boldest dream" had materialized right on my screen just as SCP had promised, and in the process, it emboldened me to write this memoir.

A French architectural magazine had featured the purchase and renovation of an impressive estate in France by an

American businessperson (my former boss) and his partner. It was a mind-boggling portrait of acquired wealth and extravagance: lush ponds stocked with trout, breathtaking landscaping, antiques, period art, an elaborate chateau, and a wine cave presumably stocked with the most expensive cabernets, chardonnays, and champagne. The feature also mentioned a favorite setting on the grounds for the proprietors to seek moments for refuge and reflection: a quaint limestone chapel nestled in a grove of cypress and olive trees.

I could've benefitted from a chapel in my backyard for refuge and reflection.

I felt a fat, juicy curse word forming in Martha's larynx. And mine.

While our RNs complained that our patients were denied the more costly equipment, therapies, and palliative medications (and I presume in HA agencies across the country), the president of the company had been searching for a slice of French real estate and an architectural legacy. I thought about him and envisioned his purchases of Louis XV chairs upholstered in rich fabric for the chateau while our patients were denied the more comfortable and medically-safer Broda chairs in their nursing homes after we were purchased by the NYC equity firm.

With that additional discovery, the true mission and vision of our hospice company was exposed. I don't care what business owners do with their hard-earned money; but in this case, their goal to use a sector of medical care to create wealth was the final straw. When I checked back to gather more information about the site, the real estate article on his website had been deleted.

A week after I started my job, our company fired the young office administrator who conducted my interview. It was an unsuspected and ugly discharge in a lengthy line of managerial dismissals during my tenure. My colleagues and I often grumbled about how the corporate headquarters seemed to retain the loyal managers and oust the competent ones.

It was sobering to realize that our hospice company existed to produce wealth for its owners, investors, and top-tier employees on the backs of the dying; my husband included. As a chaplain, I began to realize that when the description of a primary stakeholder shifts to the circling financial vultures, patients begin to fall through the cracks.

The platitude "let them eat cake" summarized the apathy toward the lower classes by the powerful of eighteenth-century France. And in our company, a similar pithy but heartless slogan was implied: "They're dying anyway, so what difference does it make?" That unspoken callousness epitomized the corporate culture by the middle of my tenure. That casual indifference to hospice care ushered in the advent of sloppy policies, lax protocols, a reduction in resources, and negligence. Our hospice owners and managers refused to see the truth and never portrayed a servant-attitude. We needed a more appropriate logo on that hillside billboard: "Hospice Take Advantage."

Many former employees from HA have shared their disdain with me. One professional, a current marketing director of an independent nonprofit hospice, summed up his encounter with our company during an interview with me: "I decided to leave HA because my values were incongruent with those of its owner. The boss obsessed about the numbers, growing the census quickly, holding down expenses to the detriment of patients, and making money. He also viewed his sales staff as commodities, easily replaced if they didn't produce big results." This employee had quit before I arrived in 2010. Our former owner must've been plotting the company's course based on his financial vision from its inception in 2004.

During the numerous careers I've enjoyed, I've learned that one quality separates authentic leadership from ineptitude: *empathy*. That one characteristic will alert potential employees and hospice consumers alike if the company should even be in the vicinity of a dying patient. The head honchos of HA and "the sentinels" they hired to safeguard the profits and generate better returns did not demonstrate an ounce of compassion for our patients, staff, or their families.

When executives, owners, investors, stockholders, or even queens do not intend to uplift humanity through their management and their three-year vision is to ransack an organization and plunder its profits, the collateral damage that ensues should not become a normal way of doing business.

There's No Place Like Home

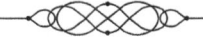

"I am not anti-hospice at all, but I think people aren't prepared for all the effort that it takes to give someone a good death at home."

Joy Johnston, Atlanta writer

In *The Wizard of Oz*, Dorothy traveled to Emerald City searching for the right place to satisfy the deepest desires of her heart. There she realized that there's really no place like home. According to a recent Kaiser Family Foundation poll, seven in ten Americans agree with Dorothy and admit they would prefer to die in the comfort of their homes. And that is the direction the health care system is moving toward, hoping to avoid unnecessary and expensive treatment at the end of life.

Millions of seniors envision their final months withering away in a nursing home with all of the inherent problems, such as inadequate staffing, the COVID pandemic still circling, the sense of isolation, and institutional decor and food. But dying at home is not all it's cracked up to be either. Too often, there aren't enough hospice staff to educate families sufficiently and oversee their attempts at care.

The die-at-home argument is persuasive. People envision a good death lying beneath a cozy coverlet and snuggling with beloved pets nestled in their own beds. Surrounded by precious mementos and lingering memories, they entertain visitors and enjoy the quiet of their own familiar space. But most of my hospice patients lived in nursing homes, contrary to public opinion that most people die at home. Many elder-care residences are beautiful, and their employees work diligently to provide comforting, cheerful, and home-like environments. But too often, those are the expensive options.

I recommend to hospice consumers that a nonprofit senior-living residence with its own independent hospice would be my first choice, instead of dying at home, if a family doesn't have the resources or time to provide round-the-clock caregiving. Hospice statistics show that the average time on service is around three weeks to seven weeks. In that case, most families can muster enough volunteers to take shifts, but even then, it can be a challenging task to provide such a demanding level of care at a stressful time.

The hospice provider gets paid around $200 or more per day per patient, whether a team member is scheduled to show up or not. Again, competent hospice providers will thoroughly educate the family and provide support for both the patient and their family, but it's so labor intensive that a lot of providers become lax. It can be daunting for untrained family members who undertake 90 percent of the hospice care at home. The system seems set up to place at-home hospice care on the backs of family caregivers while investor-owned hospice companies enjoy ever larger profits.

Johnston said that "she was surprised that her mother's hospice provider left most of the physical work to her." Families will indeed undertake the brunt of bathing, grooming, and night-shift duty. Relatives may be squeamish about giving sponge baths and changing the Depends on a confused and rebellious dementia patient. They might not realize that morphine, constipation, and inserting suppositories go hand in hand.

Unfortunately, for-profit hospice providers often view the families as the primary caregivers. I've had hospice consumers complain that in that case, "the agencies assume a more advisory role and from a distance, even in the final, intense days when family caregivers, or nurses must continually adjust morphine doses or deal with typical end-of-life issues such as bleeding or breathing trouble."

Most families don't expect the intense preoccupation with managing symptoms even under the supervision of a medical expert. Families worry about their own competency as the primary caregivers in the home instead of being totally present to their dying loved ones in their final days and hours.

Families need to understand the dynamics of hospice care. Each member of the interdisciplinary team has its own role in providing physical, emotional, and spiritual comfort; but they are only required to visit once a week unless the patient needs continuous care, more acute care, or is actively dying. That means that when the hospice RN visits, in addition to checking on the patient, he or she must also make time to educate family members about dispensing morphine and other end-of-life medications, and how to operate medical equipment.

According to a study by Citus Health in September 2020 eight out of ten family caregivers of hospice patients often claimed that hospice providers weren't giving them the immediate responses they needed in a crisis, during rapid declines, or for urgent questions.

On the other hand, the good news for at-home caregivers is that hospice delivers all of the needed medical equipment and furniture to the patient's home. Also, all companies are required to provide respite opportunities for the main caregiver, and an inpatient hospice referral for the patient—these are two of the four levels of care that all companies are required to provide for at-home caregivers. When severe symptoms cannot be handled within the home, a hospice must provide round-the-clock care in an inpatient facility for the patient. These are the many issues that consumers must clear up before they hire a provider.

Dr. Arthur Kleinman, a professor of psychiatry and anthropology at Harvard, stated on January 21, 2020: "The health-care system fails to educate and support family caregivers, who are the backbone of the nation's long-term care system. Caregivers bear too much of the burden of home hospice care."

Lessons and Insights

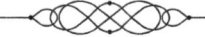

"The Divine pattern that the Spirit of God reveals is loss & renewal, and death & resurrection. There is no other way. Unfortunately, what human beings really want is resurrection without death, answers without doubt, and the conclusion without the process."

Father Richard Rohr, OFM, American Franciscan Priest

AS I LOOK BACK ON MY MINISTRY AS A HOSPICE CHAPLAIN while working for a private equity firm, I list the insights I acquired and the lessons I learned (in no particular order). Some of my insights might be embarrassingly obvious to others.

Deep down, I understood that God was always with me.

My faith is fierce.

I am not afraid to die. Jesus told us not to be afraid three hundred and sixty-five times.

I am also not afraid to take healthy risks. Life is miraculous. Go for it.

I am no longer afraid of periods of inner darkness either. Love can shine brightest there.

I try to be aware of beauty and benevolence every day.

When I lower my expectations, I feel more content.

Life is short. Do what you need to do. Don't wait.

Don't be afraid to act on behalf of the vulnerable, and for justice.

I was not my ministry or career. It was my vocation, but not my worth.

Change is constant. So I learned to concede to uncertainty.

Self-care is crucial. It's like accessing the oxygen on a flight before helping others.

We cannot love others if we don't love ourselves first. Stay healthy mentally.

I learned that you cannot help people if they don't want help.

Don't wait until a crisis to do your inner work. You will be a better partner and friend.

"Surrendering does not mean that one quits grieving what was lost; it means one accepts new circumstances and a new sense of purpose." Joan Chittister, Feminist theologian

We're all wounded, so I try to be a wounded *healer*.

Spewing toxicity into the world isn't healthy for anyone.

Mark was right. I am continuing to lead the life I was meant to live and I am happy.

It was okay not to be perfect; a constant scourge of the One (Enneagram).

I do want to end my life on earth as an enlightened person.

Periods of silence and meditation keep me grounded.

The only thing that keeps my life on track is nurturing my relationship with God.

Keep moving forward, no matter how difficult.

But I've learned that it helps to move forward on the right path. Pray to discern that path.

It helps me to stay present if I spend more time in my heart than my head.

When I'm throwing myself a "pity party," I browse through my gratitude journal.

Being around water always refreshes me and provides some serenity.

Families need to be strong advocates for their loved ones while on hospice service.

I've noticed that it was mostly women who sat vigil at the bedside of dying loved ones.

Writing this narrative took a lot of patience, sacrifice, and courage.

I have forgiven the multiple owners of Hospice Advantage for the suffering we endured under their self-serving management and unethical decision making.

And finally, as I dealt with the long hours of hospice work, middle-of-the-night patient visits, and Mark's end-stage heart failure and subsequent death, I was eventually forced to slow down and exercise self-care. Unfortunately, it takes a lot to bring me to my knees. I'm such a stubborn German.

While still in high school, I arrived home one afternoon to find a metal, circular pin on my dresser. It depicted a sloth lying on a bed of flowers. A gift from my mother. The slogan said: "Don't forget to smell the flowers." She had stood by and watched as I lived my life, even as a young teen, at a hectic pace. The curse of the first-born is a Type-A Personality; and in my case, it bordered on hypomania.

One day, I discovered this poem on *Resting* by Wendell Berry. *The sense of [resting] may come with watching a flock of cedar waxwings eating wild grapes in the top of the woods on a November afternoon. Everything they do is leisurely. They pick the grapes with curious deliberation, comb their feathers, and converse in high windy whistles. Now and then, one will fly out and back in a sort of dancing flight full of whimsical flutters and turns. They are like farmers loafing in their own fields on a Sunday. Though the waxwings have no Sundays, their days are full of sabbaths.*

I desperately want my remaining years to be full of leisurely sabbaths, like those of the cedar waxwings. Mom, I promise to dance with joy, gratitude, and a sense of whimsy. I promise to take time to "smell the flowers." I want to explore life going forward from a place of rest.

Afterword

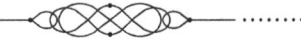

> *"[The search for] truth makes a personal, spiritual, and moral demand upon us. It hurts, it's inconvenient, and [it's time consuming]; but it's essential to our well-being."*
>
> Dr. Jacqui Lewis, Presbyterian minister, speaker, and activist

S O WHY DID I BOTHER TO SIT DOWN IN FRONT OF A SUBSTANtial hospice database in a stuffy third-floor bookstore, on a sultry day, searching for a needle in a haystack? I guess I felt compelled to at least to try to unearth what had happened at our company—for our patients, their families, and my beloved colleagues. And for Mark.

Or for that matter, what propelled me to choose to study behind the Iron Curtain during the height of the Cold War my junior year in college when friendlier cities and more accomplished music programs were available in other European cities? I guess I understood that a ten-month encounter with that period of history was a once-in-a-lifetime opportunity.

What I didn't understand at the time was that only in West Berlin, Germany, and in the Soviet-occupied spaces of postwar Europe would I have had the platform to become acquainted with injustice. Up close. I suppose that my white privilege in America was such that I needed to cross oceans to witness abuse and suffering. Living behind the Iron Curtain was a deliberate synchronization of time and place for me. Subsequently, living within blocks to the suffering of refugees and victims of violence for nine months became crucial for my preparation as a hospice chaplain.

In choosing to study in a place defined by barbed wire, concrete, guns, and the separation of families, I developed a sense of compassion that helped me to understand the suffering of John, Martha, Helen, George, Mark, and hundreds of other patients. It was in living under the constraints of the spoils of war and the scrutinizing eyes of Soviet henchmen that motivated me to be a woman of action. To be alert. To care. To look beneath the surface and uncover dead canaries wherever they may lie. To never ignore, disregard, or overlook what appears too obvious—like superficial marketing campaigns and covert missions that concealed greed. And not to take just anyone's word for the "truth" of any matter.

I could not ease people through walls of barbed wire or through dictatorships of iron-fisted hate, but I could ease them through the thin veils of death toward perfect love and mercy. I could shed light on a pastoral end-of-life movement that, yes, needed a course correction—a U-turn back to its roots—but was ultimately beautiful in its initial mission.

Maya Angelou also said, "A bird doesn't sing because it has an answer, it sings because it has a song." My work as a hospice chaplain handed me a song . . . a story. And it was just my "dumb luck" that I had been trained on how to write, read, research, and think critically. I guess I had been prepared to write this book all my life. I had no excuses. And learning about the merits of slowing down helped me to pay attention to what was right in front of me and connect the dots.

So, I wrote this narrative about a hospice company that was purchased by professional investors and the collateral damage to the human beings that got in the way.

I had never realized that an institution could be evil, in and of itself, until an RN at HA mentioned one evening at work that she felt a sense of evil in our office space.

I was the one who was in the room, on the phone, and reading the emails when the negligence, forays into criminal activity, and immoral behavior were perpetrated. The bottom line? The concept of hospice care as a medical benefit for its citizens is not the problem, but end-of-life medical care used as a vehicle to generate wealth is the problem.

PART TWO
How To Make What's Invisible, Visible

How to Find a Trustworthy Provider

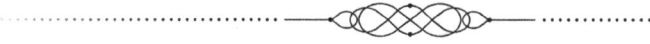

"I had always known that life was not about appetite and acquisition. In my earnest, angry, good-girl way . . . I pursued meaning."

Vivian Gornick, critic and author

I LOVE THE QUOTE I CHOSE FOR THIS CHAPTER. I AM EARNEST. I try to be a good woman. And I feel happy stepping off the curb each morning with a sense of purpose and meaning. Also, it is true that the miscarriage of justice and the exploitation of the weak and vulnerable and marginalized people does piss me off.

Navigating the large-scale industry that is hospice can be intimidating. Choosing a hospice is a crucial decision with possibly dire consequences for patients and family members if tackled in a haphazard manner. Not all hospices are equal, so it's important to get this choice right because the comfort of your loved one in the final months, weeks, and hours will depend on it. However, it's realistic to consider that as you begin your search that all institutions have their failings: the church, banking, the government, education, and medical care.

The ideal time to learn about an end-of-life partnership should be long before you need it. It should be similar to searching for the most competent and experienced surgeon, skilled lawyer, safest automobile, or well-constructed house. Hiring a hospice is an exercise in patience and research. The traumatic news of a terminal diagnosis and a life-limiting prognosis demands the companionship of a reliable hospice expert—one with pure intentions. Patients always come first.

Over 1.4 million patients receive care from a hospice organization each year, according to the Center for Disease Control and Prevention. There are over five thousand hospice providers in the US. In my metro area alone, there are seventeen hospice providers. So how does one go about finding the right hospice? The best fit? The most trustworthy?

It's important to understand that online resources for *directly* comparing the quality of hospices does not yet exist because not all hospices contribute data to the CMS. The Hospice Compare website for consumers is a tool that I've found to be incomplete, complex, time consuming, and not user-friendly. The site also conveys cautionary information about the collation of the data and the validity of the results: "this information is only *a snapshot* of [a provider's] overall quality of care." A snapshot of a slice of a mountain range does not give tourists an understanding of its scale and notable features. And if a consumer Googles "Best Hospice Care Services," links will surface to websites of any and all providers with small-print notices of caution attached: "if you ascribe to a service or provider we recommend on this site, we may earn a commission."

It's important to understand that the hospice market has changed during the last thirty years; it has transitioned from a grassroots, community-run, and independent nonprofit service to large markets of mostly for-profit corporations with a national presence and run on a proprietary basis. Hospice companies can function as part of a large national chain, operate as a subsidiary under one parent company, or as a commodity within a portfolio with other diverse business entities. Many corporations that own hospice organizations are publicly traded.

Usually hospice referrals originate with a patient's personal physician, a hospital, through a provider's own sales division, a nursing home, or through word of mouth. At the initial meeting, hospice personnel arrive with legal paperwork to enroll you or your loved one. A member of the clinical team (usually the RN, SW, or chaplain) will address your questions about hospice and typical end-of-life care.

Incidentally, every day, ten thousand senior citizens become eligible for Medicare. In 2019, 60 percent of Medicare beneficiaries died on hospice care, which amounts to around 1.5 million people.

When consumers ask me what my hospice preference was for my own parents in their final weeks, I told them I partnered with a nonprofit hospice. Nonprofit strategies for fiscal management, clinical protocols, and hospice policies are all designed for the benefit of the patient, their families, and staff. Period. No slices of the pie are plated for executives, private-equity firms, venture capitalists, banks, or stockholders. I prefer nonprofit economic enterprises because they are formed for noncommercial purposes, whether that be charitable, social, religious, scientific, or some other noble cause for humankind.

The essential first questions for the staff of a for-profit hospice provider should be: *Who owns your company? Why does your company exist? What is your primary goal for your company? Who is your primary stakeholder?* However, if prospective families asked me who owned our company in 2012, I would've given an incorrect response. None of the interdisciplinary teams were apprised that our ownership had changed. So, checking out hospice corporations on Google is a crucial step in your search. Listed here are my priorities for the hospice care of family, friends, and consumers.

1. Nonprofit inpatient residences owned by health-care systems or independent providers.
2. Religious institutions (nonprofit) that have organized hospice services in their own facilities or contract with reputable providers in the home.

3. Small, community-based for-profit hospice companies that model a nonprofit, mission-driven philosophy and practice.
4. Medium-sized for-profit companies that are not owned by professional investors.

One of the many reasons that I promote nonprofit, inpatient hospice care was the peaceful dying process both of my parents experienced.

Consumers ask me the difference between nonprofit and for-profit hospice providers. Generally, the difference has to do with purpose, goals, ownership structure, and method of generating revenue. For example, a nonprofit provider should focus primarily on a service that benefits society and whose goal places the patient as the primary stakeholder of its business.

A nonprofit company does not pay taxes to state or federal governments, so any year-end surplus must be redistributed back into the company to benefit the mission—resources for the patient. On the other hand, the mission in too many for-profit hospice companies must be to maintain a balance between generating income and serving investors, shareholders, and patients. However, as hospice has become corporatized, too many companies place owners, executives, and investors as their primary stakeholders over patients.

My chapter on vetting a hospice helps consumers determine which companies are truly aligned with a patient-first priority. Obviously, a company needs to make money to sustain its business and mission. The question is: How do they ensure an appropriate balance?

Consumers also need to understand that the "U.S. health care system is a mix of public and private, for-profit and nonprofit services. And forty percent of acute-care hospitals are for-profit." (2020 statistics released by The Commonwealth Fund Foundation).

During my research, I learned that some health care systems who advertise publicly as being "mission-driven, not-for-profit organizations" are being less than candid about the scope of their financial dealings. To be honest, I'm becoming more confused about the economic status of many hospitals and health care systems who promote themselves as not-for-profit institutions.

I recently stumbled upon a health care system that I was unaware of, but it is listed as a nonprofit hospice provider in Wisconsin. I was unaware of it because the name of its hospice division (which I was aware of) is not what they use on their website to communicate their services. During my search, a variety of articles came up describing the financial transactions over the past year of this particular Ohio-based health system. The most notable was a post written by Jim Parker on his hospice news site: "Gentiva Inked a Deal to Acquire Heartland Hospice from ProMedica (Health Care System) for $710 Million" (2/27/2023). The transaction was expected to close in the second quarter of this past year.

Heartland's parent company is ProMedica which also includes a network of 13 hospitals and other healthcare services. What is a parent company? It's a corporation, also known as a holding company, that controls a subsidiary company (like Heartland Hospice) owning a majority stake and influencing its direction. The reasons for forming a parent company include diversification, capital access, tax benefits, dumping assets, and expansion through acquisitions.

Gentiva Hospice is a portfolio company of the private equity firm Clayton, Dubilier & Rice (CDR) and Humana Inc. So, from my calculations, with the acquisition of Heartland Hospice, Gentiva should number about 34,000 patients and rank as one of the largest for-profit providers in the US. Coincidentally, while the Heartland Hospice Agencies have been purportedly sold to Gentiva Hospice services, ProMedica will come up when a hospice consumer puts Heartland into the search engine. They seem to be sharing a single identity at this point. Parent companies should not be advertisers for one of their specific business entities. Imagine if the parent company of for-profit VITAS Hospice, Roto-Rooter (Chemed), was the primary advertiser of their hospice company. Plumbing services or end-of-life care? I can still sing their catchy advertising jingle. However, it's confusing for consumers. Consumers deserve full transparency.

Dr. Cicely Saunders started hospice to focus only on the patient and their families in a pastoral setting. Money never entered into her vision. The original purpose of hospice has been buried under the weight of multiple acquisitions and mergers and parent companies and stockholders and financial opportunists in the senior care market.

Why should hospice consumers be concerned? Who cares what the actual name of the hospice is? Who cares that Hospice Advantage is now Compassus, and Gentiva emerged from Kindred, and Heartland Hospice will soon officially be under the wing of Gentiva? I could cite many more examples. When hospice first began, it didn't need the support of "parents" or private equity firms to deliver stellar care.

So why should you be concerned? Because when huge and ongoing financial transactions are a priority, your family members are not. In fact, as hospice has been increasingly commercialized, their care has been compromised.

An example of poor care is an event whereby an infusion of morphine is needed to stem severe pain, and the equipment is not available until the next day. Poor care is when a company does not have enough staff on third shift and a family member must sit up all night to administer opioid injections every hour instead of resting in the knowledge that their loved one is comfortable and is being monitored by a professional during a change in condition. Family members need compassionate relief and sleep as well. Poor care is when oxygen is needed and the equipment is delivered in disrepair.

It is not the fault of the staff or the hospice model that healthcare systems that advertise as not-for-profit economies pour millions into the pockets of their CEOs as annual compensation. This is the type of research that consumers can do in thirty minutes to ascertain the true mission of any health care company.

Be wary of the actual goal of a company with a hospice division and not the content on their shiny billboards. Not all health care systems and hospitals are truly nonprofit as advertised. Let's promote the institutions that mirror the original hospice model.

A fine example of excellent nonprofit, in-patient care was what my father experienced in his final days. He progressed from assisted living to residential hospice care. He had end-stage liver cancer. Upon arrival, we paid his room and board because Medicare only pays for the hospice care. At certain levels of care, Medicare kicks in for room and board as well.

After two weeks, my dad's vital signs became abnormal and he had difficulty swallowing. The staff had trouble clearing his airway, his pain had increased, and he could no longer get out of bed. He was within days of dying. I remember how frightening it seemed, and my family had a professional hospice staff just steps away.

Our RN tried a variety of medications to clear his airway, but the staff finally succumbed to suctioning him with the equipment built into the wall above his bed. The convenience of round-the-clock pain management, palliative care to ease other uncomfortable symptoms, and end-of-life medical equipment in the building was so comforting to us.

I thought about families dealing with all of this in their cleared-out dining rooms. We never had to wait in desperation for a provider to return a phone call or email. There was no fretting about correct dosages or how to address a sudden change in condition. We simply pressed the call button and hospice experts hustled down the hall. The wonderful staff of ProHealth AngelsGrace Hospice delivered end-of-life medical care around-the-clock, and we concentrated on loving our father with the time he had left.

Qualities of a Reputable Provider

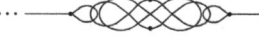

"While many for-profit hospices do good work, structuring end-of-life care as a machine for revenue generation poses risks to both clinicians and patients."

Dr. Nathan A. Gray, MD, assistant professor of medicine at Johns Hopkins University, hospice and palliative medicine consultant, cartoonist on life and medical issues

FAMILIES NEED TO ASK THEMSELVES WHAT TYPE OF HOSPICE provider they want to be in a relationship with as they prepare to leave this world. I ask consumers who call me with hospice complaints to tell me if the company they partnered with was for-profit or nonprofit. Most have no clue. It's a critical question. To have a good chance at a five-star dying experience, prospective hospice consumers need to discern the higher purpose of a hospice provider. Consumers need to understand the economic structure of a hospice because more upfront legwork will be needed if it's a for-profit provider.

The core values of a hospice company have nothing to do with their eye-catching logo, brand, or glitzy advertising. The mission and vision statements should be genuine goals of an organization's internal infrastructure. The mission statement defines the company's business, its objectives, and their approach to reaching those objectives. A vision statement describes the desired future position of the company. The elements of these two statements combined provide a declaration of the company's purposes, goals, and values. Consumers deserve to know a company's long-term objectives because that vision will define who their primary stakeholders are. Investors or patients.

Hospice consumers have many choices. It is critical to search for a provider owned by people who want to elevate humanity through their financial dealings; not all for-profit companies are profiteers. There are many who do protect the dignity of the dying, and I list two models here.

Mountain Home Health Care and Hospice in Taos, New Mexico, is a licensed 501(c)(3) nonprofit hospice provider that is transparent about its finances online and lists its purpose, not its logo, in its advertising. A nine-member board of directors governs the company that is built on a foundation of a strong bond with local doctors and Taos County Hospitals. Its mission statement online states that its deep passion for hospice care and its respect for the Taos community fuel delivery of outstanding care.

Badger Hospice is a for-profit newcomer to southeastern Wisconsin. One owner of the local company is Barbara Horstmeyer. She believed that hospice was becoming too commercial, so she gathered like-minded health-care providers who shared her concern and vision and founded Badger Hospice, LLC in 2016.

Badger RN Joanne Swanson added: "As a nurse and former owner of a specialty care residence for older adults, I've had the opportunity to witness and experience hospice services by many different providers over the years, and it is clear that not all hospices are equal."

The CEO of Badger Hospice, Laura Kukowski, understands that "a for-profit business must balance a payroll and meet expenses, while at the same time, sustain the mission of good patient care." What is so vastly different in this for-profit hospice is that the CEO is a hands-on manager. It is a small-enough operation that she knows the staff, patients, and families. The staff says she has built an in-office culture of transparency, honesty, and respect. She has organized nursing shifts to maintain a safe and healthy work-life balance. Contented employees are a sign of a healthy hospice provider.

Kukowski realizes that a staff treated with dignity and fairness remains loyal, which lends itself to consistent protocols, which leads to greater family satisfaction, and a higher quality of patient care. Badger Hospice is a for-profit company that leads with a commitment to excellent care and places its patients and families as their primary stakeholders. This is why I've been careful not to paint all for-profit hospices with a broad brush. There are very good for-profit hospices, but you need to ask the right questions to locate them.

It would be refreshing to see a company respond to questions about its mission and vision with a philosophy such as the "triple bottom line" (TBL). A TBL philosophy for a hospice is an ideology that considers the parceling out of net income (through resources) to patients and employees first. And a component of that philosophy is that the planet is not harmed in the process (if that applies). This isn't a new concept.

When John Elkington, an authority on corporate responsibility and sustainable development, first mentioned TBL in the mid-1990s, he also laid the groundwork for defining the social impacts of a company's practices and activities. In the hospice industry, those social impacts would include the physical comfort and moral dignity of each patient, and the sufficient education and support of those families who have loved ones dying in their homes.

As a hospice professional, I wanted to work for a company that operated ethically, acted with integrity, and cared about the people who worked for it; a company that focused on building a culture of "we" rather than a culture of "me." I had thought that I was hired by such a company when I began working at HA. And in the beginning, it appeared to be real. But in time, I found out that I was inadvertently helping to conceal a change in mission that was not good for our patients.

It's imperative to understand that the goals of nonprofit hospices and smaller for-profit agencies are that their strategies, financial management, clinical protocols, and policies are instituted to benefit patients and their families. The scale is balanced in favor of the patients and their families.

Incidentally, the definition of a nonprofit company is that it is formed to carry out a noncommercial purpose whether that be charitable, social, religious, scientific, or some other noble cause for humankind. That is the reason I encourage families to seek nonprofit providers first. As well, research shows that nonprofit providers outperform for-profit providers in hospice care.

Consumers ask me why the preferred option for hospice care shouldn't be for-profit as they have a lot more money at their disposal to support patient care. The current statistics do support that logical theory; the average profit margins for nonprofit agencies hover around 5.9 percent, compared to near 20 percent among for-profit agencies. However, what is happening in the corporate sector of hospice is that the incentive to cut the quality of care to serve the bottom line is high; so patients are not reaping the additional benefits from the increased capital.

As a chaplain, my hospice colleagues had to educate me on how that worked. They explained that the bundled-payment structure meant that the main source of profit for these corporations is the difference between the *actual cost* of patient care provided to hospices by Medicare and private insurance and the *fixed daily payments.*

For example, if the payment to a hospice is around $200 per day (per patient), and the hospice only spends $100 on each patient, then the corporation makes money. If I understand this correctly, it seems as if taxpayers (through the CMS hospice entitlements) are paying private investors to get rich.

The statistics show that "on average, *for-profit hospices spent less per day on patient care*; were less likely to provide visits in the last few days of life; employed fewer skilled staff, and were less likely to provide care at a dedicated hospice facility for crisis management."

In the next chapter, I list the quintessential questions for selecting a quality hospice. You will not find these questions on the Internet, on a hospice website, or at a physician's office. While the widely-disseminated clinical information by the hospice industry is valuable, it will not help consumers discern the true motives or core values of a large for-profit provider.

My tools will help consumers discern which for-profit companies place their patients as their authentic stakeholders. But why is the list so extensive? Because I had acquired so much pertinent information from my hospice ministry, consumer advocacy work, and research into hospice ownership statistics—the inventory of helpful questions exploded. That catalogue of information will educate you on the for-profit hospice market. These questions are suggestions, so educate yourself, and utilize the ones that are most helpful to you.

The easiest way to go behind the window dressing (glitzy advertising, pompous promises, and polished image) is to do an online search of its financial acquisition-and-merger history, the specifics of its economic structure, history of ownership, if it's publicly held, its size, and the investment groups involved. All of this information is public and easy to find.

Most of the data you need to vet a for-profit hospice is listed on the websites of the equity firms and corporations that own a particular hospice company. For example, if you Google any for-profit company you can download reams of pertinent information.

The business side of hospice is not necessarily a dirty enterprise. But there needs to be adequate government oversight so the industry can remain true to its pastoral roots.

Behind the Window Dressing

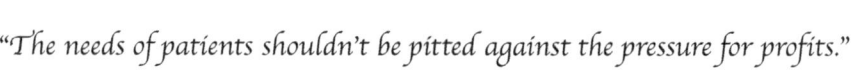

"The needs of patients shouldn't be pitted against the pressure for profits."
Frank M., Hospice Advantage marketing representative

THE QUESTIONS THAT I HAVE FORMULATED FOR THIS CHAPTER come from my experiences working at HA and speaking to disgruntled families when I worked as a hospice consumer advocate. These questions are tools that can help you determine whether a company is poorly managed, short-staffed, negligent, or one who places investors as their primary stakeholders. These tools may help uncover a few gnarly issues or may pull up a dirty, dead-as-a-doornail canary (from a toxic hospice environment).

No medical care is perfect. All hospices face challenges, regardless of economic structure, but these tools will help you determine if the hospice advertisements on billboards, pamphlets, and websites correlate to good medicine. It won't be simple. After all, the practice of bad management in senior care and in hospice management has largely escaped government notice for years.

These chapters on vetting hospice providers will assist consumers in weeding out the companies that covet large profits to the detriment of patient care. At the same time, I hope the for-profit hospice providers that serve patients with integrity will be recognized and rewarded.

The following questions will give you insider information about the business side of hospice for interviews with for-profit providers. For-profit hospice companies do not advertise their economic status on their website, but trustworthy for-profit hospices will be happy to answer questions about their priorities and economic structure during an interview.

This list of educational questions is only a guide.

1. Who owns the for-profit hospice?
    - A multi-industry corporation that also owns hospice agencies.
    - A hospice company with a national chain of providers.
    - A private equity firm.
    - A bank.
    - An insurance provider.
    - A retail corporation.
    - A family.
    - Venture capitalists and stockholders.
2. What is the ownership history?
3. Is the company in the process of selling to an equity firm, or in the middle of an acquisition or merger? To whom? (Bigger is not better.)
4. If the agency is a part of a national hospice chain, ask about the company's geographical area, number of employees, and census.
5. What is the company's financial vision for the next four years?
6. What was your mission when you started this company? What is it today?
7. How do you execute your mission? Give examples.
8. What is the patient-to-RN ratio? (A former RN administrator said twelve patients per RN would be the highest ratio, but HA had as many as seventeen patients per RN at one point.)

9. What percentage of your profit is distributed to patient care, staff salaries, benefits, and training?
10. How do you increase your census?
11. What partnerships have you formed within the community?
12. Do you post your family satisfaction surveys on your website?
13. Have you ever been cited for negligence or fraud? A lot of companies are not cited, but should be.
14. After signing a contract with a provider, if a family finds that the service is not meeting its needs can they ask to be discharged and search for another provider? (Yes.)
15. How does your company measure success?
16. As a for-profit company, how do you balance a business with excellence in care?
17. Who do you consider the primary stakeholders of your company? Explain. Who would be second? Third?
18. What type of technology do you use to communicate with families and staff?

Additional questions for both nonprofit and for-profit providers.

1. What is the five-year staff turnover rate for hospice RNs and CNAs? (The turnover rate for 2021 was almost 27 percent.)
2. What is your yearly patient-discharge rate? (In 2017, one in five patients were discharged from hospice care. A high discharge rate is not good.)
3. How many additional requests for patient documentation do you get from Medicare?
4. Are all of your RNs certified in hospice care?
5. Do your cancer patients receive palliative chemotherapy in the hospital for comfort, if needed?
6. Do you have enough staff to provide "continuous nursing care" if a patient experiences a severe medical crisis?

7. How do you staff for third shift and weekends? How large is your service area?
8. Do you allow palliative treatment in the hospital if it increases the patient's quality of life? Our company did not allow a hospital admission for comfort care. Hospice never allows a hospital admission for curative care.
9. Inquire about additional services: pet therapy, speech and physical therapy, doula services, massage, and music therapy. All hospices must offer grief counselling, respite care, and train volunteers.

Questions for hospice care in nursing homes.

1. Do you educate nursing home staff on different types of pain management and the hospice philosophy? (Often, hospice care is only as effective and consistent as the excellence and professionalism of the nursing facility it contracts with.)
2. What is the quality of your relationships with skilled nursing facilities (SNF)? (The SNF remains the primary caregiver of hospice patients. The skilled-nursing staff and the hospice team must communicate well and work together for the benefit of the patient.)
3. Will my loved one keep the same interdisciplinary team while receiving care?
4. What is the average frequency of visits for each patient by the clinical team after the initial signup and before the actively-dying stage?
5. Does the patient's physician or hospice medical director follow the patient?
6. What happens to the patient's medications once hospice care is started?
7. What are the protocols you utilize to manage unresolved pain issues?

Questions for hospice care at home.

1. How many hours of end-of-life education do you offer to families? What is the ratio of clinical visits versus family caregiving hours?
2. Where do you score on the family surveys for your at-home hospice service?
3. How long does it typically take an RN to reach a patient after an initial notification for help? On second and third shift? (Often it depends on the distance of the service area.)
4. How long does it take for a family to receive advice, equipment, and assistance?
5. Is it appropriate for a family to call a rescue squad for help while on hospice? (The answer should be never.)
6. Do you provide respite care for at-home caregivers. How long?
7. What facility do you use for respite care?
8. What facility do you use for 24/7 care for symptoms that can't be managed at home?

The main reason I list these questions is that the ethos of a hospice business—its values, principles, and practices—could be uncovered through the responses you receive and through the research you gather. Forthright answers can affirm the authenticity of a company's logo, brand, and advertising; and exposing the true mission and motivations of a company can only help patients and their families.

If responses to your questions aren't answered to your satisfaction in an interview (which many might not be), then proceed with an in-depth search of the company's financial history online. For example, if you Google the owner of VITAS Hospice, the following information will pop up: the parent organization (Chemed Corporation) along with the name Comfort Care Holdings. The website or an article will detail the history of the mergers and acquisitions of VITAS, and the profiles of the company executives will be listed alongside the company's net worth and stock prices.

The net revenue for VITAS in the first quarter of 2021, $316 million, will also be listed. Also, you can Google the current CEO of the company and his background. What you might realize by now is that the true mission of a hospice company will be revealed by its size, the complexity of its financial holdings, public offerings, and the acquisition and merger trail of its owners.

Is it impossible to receive good hospice care in a large hospice company or from a corporation? Not necessarily, but I'd rather err on the side of a company whose designated mission is "patients first" rather than under the pressure of "investors first." Also, it's crucial for families to understand that they are not required to use the hospice services that have a contract with a particular nursing home; or a hospice under contract with their Medicare insurance, for that matter. They can sign with any provider in their area.

As a consumer, if your eyes are glazing over at this lengthy list of questions and you are short on time, relegate your search to only nonprofit providers (I list the nonprofit providers in Wisconsin at the end of the book), or community-oriented for-profit companies like for-profit Badger Hospice and Independent Rainbow Hospice in Southeastern Wisconsin. Again, a strong endorsement for a particular hospice by a friend or family member is one of the best referrals.

PART THREE

Helping Hospice Return
To Its Roots

Dying for Dollars

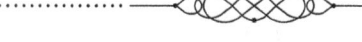

"We are imperfect mortal beings, aware of that mortality, even as we push it away."

Joan Didion, The Year of Magical Thinking.

I WANT TO STRESS HOW IMPORTANT IT IS TO UNDERSTAND THE difference between nonprofit and for-profit providers. And at the same time, consumers should realize there is a difference in the mission between small, community-oriented for-profit providers, and those of corporations owned by investors or publicly-traded on the stock market.

In the book *Changing The Way We Die,* journalists Himmel and Smith describe the evolution of how the hospice movement grew into a full-fledged financial industry deliberately engineered to make money. They tell the story of a United Methodist minister, Rev. Hugh Westbrook who invented the very idea of the corporate hospice when he and a couple of partners opened the first for-profit program in Dallas, in 1984—right after the Medicare law he was instrumental in crafting began to pay for hospice services.

In 1993, hospice became a nationally guaranteed benefit under President Clinton's health care reform (NHPCO, 2016). Over the next two decades, the reverend grew the company into VITAS Innovative Hospice Care, a pioneer in the hospice movement since

1978, and the nation's leading provider of end-of-life care. Authors Himmel and Smith concluded that Westbrook proved the unthinkable: A business could make a fortune caring for dying people.

He cashed out to Roto-Rooter, a publicly-traded company and a longtime VITAS investor. Roto-Rooter already owned about 25 percent of VITAS when it acquired the rest of the company in a $406 million deal in 2004. Rev. Westbrook walked away with $200 million in his pocket.

The corporate world was watching. Everyone wanted a piece of that booming industry. Apparently, someone I would come to make the acquaintance of was also watching from the sidelines—my former hospice employer. He started Hospice Advantage the same year Westbrook pocketed the $200 million.

Investor-owned hospice companies grow through classic business strategies: cost controls, volume purchasing, efficiencies that come with size, recapitalization, and marketing. "Rev. Westbrook also hired marketing representatives, a job title that did not previously exist in the hospice field until the 1990s. Their initial role was to persuade doctors, hospitals, and nursing homes to make referrals to their own hospice companies." A competition soon surged among providers and conflicts of interest confused families. Even worse, no one questioned the quality of patient care amidst all this collaboration.

In the next eight years, the industry changed dramatically. A wave of mergers, acquisitions, and investments made hospice another Wall Street commodity, with one goal: to maximize returns. "Roto-Rooter kept its hospice operations under the VITAS name, but rebranded the corporate parent as Chemed Corp. The name had a ring of scientific authority and did not call to mind clogged drains."

Now under pressure to please stockholders with ever-increasing returns each quarter, VITAS Hospice embarked on a fast track to growth. It bought smaller hospices, opened new ones, and marketed aggressively to doctors. It served a daily census of 18,050 and reported nearly $316 million in patient revenue in 2021. Incidentally,

Kevin J. McNamara, Chemed President and CEO (since 2001), earns $10,019,800 annually. He owns Chemed stock worth about $62,773,905. The estimated net worth of Mr. McNamara is at least $167.53 million as of August 2022. VITAS became the shining example of how to make money with the end-of-life medical market.

No wonder hospice beckoned owners, executives, private equity, banks, and venture capitalists. There was a lot of money to be made amidst an enormous aging population and the increased demand for senior services. Baby boomers have had a significant impact on the demographics of the US population and the markets that serve them.

Trey Andrews, an associate at the McGuire Woods Consulting Firm, LLC, and co-author of a report on investments in senior care industries for an article in *Hospice News* on January 16, 2020, cited other criteria for such interest: Strong and sophisticated management teams in the middle markets of hospice care, the availability of smaller hospice companies and single-location providers for consolidation, and prime geography (investors are attracted to large areas with a high density of seniors and growing trends in that elderly demographic). Think of The Villages, a 57-square-mile planned senior community in Central Florida where one hundred and thirty-eight-thousand adults live.

A senior oasis and a hospice haven for investors.

"Service diversification is another key trend that is attracting investors," said Jim Parker, editor of *Hospice News*. "It is of tremendous financial benefit for a corporation to offer a 'suite' of continuous senior-care services starting with home healthcare and progressing to a comprehensive integrated-care model delivered in one complex." From independent living to assisted living to skilled nursing to memory care to hospice care to the grave. A neat, packaged concierge of care for those advancing in years.

Some folks refer to this slow progression of increased care as "the stairway to heaven." Private equity firms are in business to buy, grow, and sell companies. Any and all companies. Equity firms provide capital and build businesses through investments, expertise in business strategy, finance, marketing, and shrewd management.

Between 2010 and 2019, private-equity investment in senior care rose. But hospice consultants in the industry admitted to me that it was difficult to gauge how many investment firms were involved in the hospice market because the sales, acquisitions and mergers do not have to be made public, like nursing homes must. But according to a 2021 study, the approximate number of hospice agencies owned by private equity soared from 106 of a total of 3,162 hospices in 2011, to 409 of 5,615 operating in 2019.

Journalists Himmel and Smith cited the gross amount of money that was changing hands in their book. "For example, an undisclosed Salt Lake City-based PE firm purchased Comfort Hospice in Portland, Oregon, for $20 million. The firm owned thirty-one hospices throughout the western United States. Comfort Hospice earned nearly $8.3 million in annual revenues. Such numbers helped drive the dizzying pace of acquisitions in a field that had always prided itself on local autonomy and deep community roots."

Managing Partner Cory Mertz of the Mertz Taggart Home Care and Hospice Merger and Acquisition Report for Q4 in 2021 said, "Private equity continues to see long-term opportunity in the home health, hospice, and home care sub-sectors—and they continue to have vast stockpiles of cash they're looking to deploy. There were at least 166 large transactions that took place in corporate America worth over $1 billion and the hospice M&A market is 'as hot as it's ever been' with millions of dollars changing hands."

Transactions in the hospice market by corporate America and their investors has been hot, but the word of fraudulent and negligent hospice care was reaching law firms and the press. During this period, the Department of Justice sued many hospice providers for gaming the Medicare benefit for reimbursements for patient care. It's important to note that many senior-living residences are not-for-profit.

Critics argued that private equity should not be in the senior medical field. Ultimately, a private equity firm's commitment is to its investors and not necessarily to its patients or employees, which also means that workers may not always get the resources they need to do their jobs well if a firm reduces their operational budget which is what happened in our company.

Skeptics included James Carey, executive director of admissions of the Association of Independent Doctors, who outlined concerns in the 2018 *MarketWatch* report, "Large hospice corporations are in it for profit. Americans are going to pay for it, either with their health, lives, finances, or all of the above. And, I would add, with their suffering."

He was right.

Weak Oversight Breeds Neglect

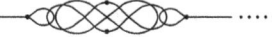

"End-of-life care deserves continued development and vigilance, and we have to erect guardrails and raise standards for all hospice providers."

Dr. Nathan A. Gray

NOBODY WANTS TO DIE. BUT DEATH IS INEVITABLE; SO THEN, no one wants to die badly. Good hospice care offers the best hope for dying well and living fully until we do. Doula workers tell me that their "goal is to restore death to its sacred place in the celebration of life." Tasks of good hospice care are three-fold: appropriate palliative care, attentive pastoral practice, and most important, timely pain management.

As a result, consumers need to understand the revelations highlighted in the July 2019 report released by the Department of Health and Human Services (HHS). The Office of Inspector General (OIG) is the oversight division of that federal agency aimed at preventing inefficient or unlawful operations in medical care. It investigated complaints of fraud, waste, and abuse within the hospice industry in 2016. The fissures in hospice care had grown wider and deep enough that even Congress and the cabinet–level branch of the US federal government had registered alarm.

HHS has been at the forefront of the nation's efforts to regulate medical programs administered by the Centers of Medicare and

Medicaid (CMS). A majority of its resources go to oversight of programs that affect the country's most vulnerable citizens. It develops initiatives and distributes funds and grants to help the healthcare industry and educate the public so people can protect themselves against negligent care.

The graying of America, coupled with the commercialization of the hospice benefit, has transformed hospice from a mission of mercy into a multi-billion-a-year healthcare enterprise. Every sector of society has been preparing for an aging world. Consequently, senior care coupled with the hospice market is expected to grow into a $550 billion-a-year industry by 2024.

It is this mind-numbing reality that has propelled corporations and professional investors to see the money-making potential of the aging population. The entry of Corporate America and private investment into the hospice industry in the last twenty years has ushered in a competitive financial equation that directly affects how hospice care is managed and practiced. The fact that hospices have become big business for private-equity firms is raising concerns about the quality of end-of-life care.

Regardless of economic structure, all hospices must meet specific federal requirements, carry state licenses, and hold Medicare certifications (if CMS is responsible for reimbursing patient treatment). Not all hospice providers are certified by Medicare and Medicaid. At least one-third of providers in the United States are independently owned.

To promote compliance, the CMS relies on state agencies and accreditation organizations to monitor hospices. As part of this process, registered nurses go into hospices in surveyor roles to evaluate medical records, family evaluations, clinical documentation, and to register complaints; however, they are not trained to go beneath the surface. They report what they see and what the agency documents.

Hospice providers have the option to undergo an accreditation process that tries to ensure that they meet or exceed current standards. There are three large accreditation organizations for hospice systems in the United States: Accreditation Commission for Health Care, Inc., Community Health Accreditation Program (CHAP), and the Joint Commission on the Accreditation of Healthcare Organizations.

One would think that supplemental accreditation would be essential for credibility to those charged with the care and comfort of hospice patients. However, as of 2015, only 40 percent of hospice providers had met the criteria. There are no public statistics on current accreditations.

The accreditation process for hospice facilities involves national standards but is often administered by the states. That is baffling. Because hospice is a medical business, standardized assessments are crucial to giving families the peace of mind that the provider invests in the highest caliber of care.

I find it troubling that a provider can be a certified and licensed agency, but not belong to a national or state hospice association that provides ongoing training and resources to maintain quality. The lack of ongoing training for hospice clinicians was also noted in the OIG report. The agency I worked for did not provide ongoing training.

While a supplemental accreditation should provide an extra guarantee of excellence and raise the reputation of a specific hospice, it can also prove misleading. Consumers need to be wary. For example, when I worked for Hospice Advantage, they were granted certification by Community Health Accreditation Partner (CHAP). CHAP accreditation demonstrates that home health, palliative care, or hospice programs meet the industries highest standards for care. But HA still gamed the system, gouged the CMS benefit, took shortcuts, and—in the process—harmed patients. Fraudulent practices and other negligence escaped the scrutiny of surveyors. We operated comfortably—just under the radar.

Without knowing the background, a typical consumer will assume that with all of this licensing, certification, and additional accreditation by providers, all hospices would be trustworthy. But the government falls short of ensuring compliance. On July 9, 2019, *Kaiser Health News* (a nonprofit news service committed to healthcare policy) noted that "the OIG Report took CMS to task for what it described as years of weak oversight and enforcement."

David Stevenson, director of health policy and education at Vanderbilt University in the College of Public Health, concurs, saying: "Hospice oversight is minimal." Stevenson added that the Federal Centers for Medicare and Medicaid Services "does not have immediate sanctions at its disposal like fines or installing temporary management for non-compliant providers."

In response to the 2019 OIG Report, the National Hospice and Palliative Care Organization stated: "Any hospice provider who fails to be fully compliant with all regulations and standards of good practice and is unwilling to provide the highest quality of care *should not be in the business of caring for the dying and their loved ones.*"

It is not hard for a hospice provider to circumvent these apparent "safeguards" that accompany licensing and accreditation. One problem with the current system used to survey agencies is that the certification process requires an *"open internal review"* of maintenance structures, protocols, policies, and complaints. This arrangement is a means to ease assessment visits by accrediting organizations.

In other words, the federal and state evaluation systems cannot handle the surveys of thousands of hospice providers. Therefore, this type of self-review system is designed to leave the fine-grain analysis of policy and practice up to the individual hospice-service provider. This is one explanation for how the fertile ground for neglect was sowed.

Disingenuous hospice providers will not blow the whistle on their own incompetence in front of families or to the state and federal surveying agencies. And when these providers have been confronted with questionable practices, negligence, or outright fraud, I've watched administrators circle the company wagons and the conversations descend into a she-said, he-said scenario. No employee wants to get fired; no business wants to get cited; no provider wants a bad reputation; and no owner and their investors want to lose money.

This makes it difficult to expose an ignoble provider: A state surveyor can only uncover so much without the supplemental information provided by the hospice. Incidentally, in the findings proposed by the OIG in 2019, a recommendation was included with the report "to strengthen the provider survey process."

A second source of difficulty is that CMS also relies on posthumous family surveys to monitor hospice providers. When I started working in bereavement in 2010, there was no national survey for families. The Strategic Healthcare Program hadn't begun to administer the Consumer Assessment of a Healthcare Provider's Hospice Survey until September 1, 2014.

Nevertheless, no one can underestimate the value of personal experience for determining the credibility of anything.

The US Government Sounds an Alarm

"An important step [to give hospice consumers confidence] will be to achieve greater transparency in public reporting on hospice ownership."

Authors Robert Tyler Braun, PhD; Mark Aaron Unruh
PhD; and Daniel G. Stephenson PhD

THE REPORT FROM THE OFFICE OF INSPECTOR GENERAL ON July 3, 2019, was based on an analysis of data from state agencies and accreditation organizations from 2012 through 2016 from *all* of the 4,000-plus Medicare-certified hospices. Independent hospice providers were not included in the study.

The report found that "the *majority* of US hospice providers that provide end-of-life care had *at least* one deficiency, meaning they failed to meet one or more of the Medicare requirements." No medical provider is perfect, so how serious are the deficiencies? How prevalent? Do hospice consumers need to worry? The OIG analysis of Medicare-covered hospice services—provided to 1.4 million beneficiaries at a cost of $16.7 billion in 2016 alone—from 2006 to 2016 found that more than 85 percent had a deficiency in the quality of the care they provided, while about 20 percent had a serious deficiency (in some cases, it meant that the health and safety of beneficiaries may be in jeopardy).

Many recipients were left in "unecessary pain for many days"; Families were not given crucial information about their loved one's care; and hospices were overbilling Medicare "hundreds of millions of dollars."

But OIG's specific examples illustrated the worst abuse most vividly: amputations stemming from neglected infections; maggots infiltrating dirty feeding tubes; broken bones from being dropped; poorly maintained equipment; uncontrolled pain and sexual abuse. These incidences of extreme negligence and utter incompetence that shocked the industry and garnered most of the media attention were isolated and occurred in a small sampling of providers—the bottom-feeders of the industry.

However, it is important to underscore four other notable characteristics of the report. First, it acknowledges that not all hospice providers in the country were surveyed—only the bulk of those certified by Medicare. About twenty-four hundred providers were not involved in the survey. Therefore, the percentage of providers operating at an "unacceptable level" is higher than the 20 percent reported.

Second, the report highlighted that none of the hospices with severe deficiencies faced serious consequences and, sadly, are still operating. Third, the investigation was completed in 2016 and the report, with its recommendations for improvement, was not released until July 2019. Therefore, those deficiencies of varying degrees continued to exist for those years. Fourth, the report revealed that for-profit agencies were more likely to have grievances than nonprofits. That is a logical deduction, as about 80 percent of hospices are structured to make profits.

In addition to the more blatant examples of abuse cited by the study, a variety of "secondary deficiencies" were also listed, including: "improper vetting of staff, inadequate quality control, deficient assessment of incoming patients, and substandard internal communication protocols."

These "secondary" deficiencies, while seemingly less alarming, were buried in headlines beneath the more shocking revelations; but, in my estimation, those inadequacies were far more damning because they corresponded to what is fundamental for good hospice care. Other weaknesses that had been documented were poor care planning, mismanagement of aide services, and substandard staff training. Again, these deficiencies are far from marginal—they are precisely the fault lines from which patient discomfort, a poor quality of life, and inadequate pain management stem.

Those are the primary tasks a hospice is in business to get right. Most importantly, implementation of the best clinical practice is how good care is assembled, disseminated, and sustained. This is critical. Options like pet therapy, music therapy, weighted lap blankets, and legacy planning are wonderful; but, in the scheme of things, those are ancillary services.

Upon the release of the eye-opening report, there was an uproar in the hospice community by many practitioners and hospice trade organizations that seemed more preoccupied with the media damage inflicted on the hospice reputation than by the actual harm inflicted on patients. Were the reports covered by the media incorrect? No. Hyped? No. The facts were simply shocking.

The slide toward poor performance in certain sectors of the industry was an ethical failing, but defensiveness about the report risked it becoming a moral one if the deficiencies were discounted and the subsequent recommendations went unheeded. The hospice industry and the government faced a reckoning.

I believe many hospice clinicians and consumers underestimated the real ramifications of the results of that report. It wasn't the gross negligence and shocking mistreatment (maybe even bordering on criminality) of a small minority of providers that merited the attention-grabbing headlines, it was the "secondary" deficiencies that truly would threaten hospice patients going forward.

How do we rightfully expose the providers who deliver substandard hospice care without tarnishing the reputation of hospice in general? We do not want to frighten prospective families from pursuing the hospice benefit, but we do need to arm them with facts and investigative tools for their search for trustworthy companies until the government can catch up with its oversight. The mantra for each hospice consumer should be, *learn what I need to know before I need to know it.*

Indeed, we need to look honestly at what the hospice experience has become; for many, it is wonderful but for too many families it is disheartening. If billions of dollars of capital from private equity investors and venture capitalists is pouring into the for-profit hospice industry, bad hospice care does not stem from the lack of financial resources. The problem lies in how those resources have been allocated.

State surveyors and national accreditation vendors are not trained to examine the business side of hospice. But the federal government has a fundamental responsibility to ensure that the billions of tax dollars that pay for hospice services are well spent and pay for the highest quality of care.

The Department of Health and Human Services was not the only agency or sector that had been looking into concerns about hospice care. Already triggered by media reports in 2014 about the aggressive enrollment practices and deficient care in the for-profit hospice sector, President Obama signed The Impact Act to bolster hospice oversight.

As well, The Institute of Medicine Report, *Dying in America,* concluded that "the provision of end-of-life care in the United States required substantial changes." The report "outlined several challenges that faced hospice and threatened its long-run viability, including the shortcomings of its static approach to patient eligibility and per diem payment methods." That was in 2015.

And finally, the Assistant Secretary for Planning and Evaluation released a report in 2018 that tracked the impact of ownership changes to the quality of hospice care (the secretary is the principal advisor to the US Department of HHS). That report highlighted disturbing trends within the for-profit sector related to the proliferation of large-chain providers. However, if anyone who could actually do something was paying attention, there was no implementation.

David G. Stevenson, PhD, wrote about the impact of ownership on hospice service way back on April 30, 2016. He cautioned that *"few analyses of hospice care are based on the role of a hospice's parent company or its investors."*

Sadly, the substantial improvements called for in the hospice industry have been slow to materialize. So, on March 29, 2022, the *Los Angeles Times* broke another heartbreaking hospice story. Its article exposed a "large-scale organized effort to defraud federal end-of-life care programs in Los Angeles County, putting vulnerable patients at risk of harm. Auditors blamed a rapid boom in the number of hospice startups, and the state's loosely-regulated hospice industry for the quality-of-care deficiencies."

The report went on to uncover "fraudulent billing to the CMS and the apparent use of stolen identities of medical personnel to obtain hospice licenses. Hospice agencies in Los Angeles County likely overbilled CMS by $105 million in 2019, alone." At taxpayer expense. These same companies sought licensure renewals and were approved, essentially placing patients at "risk of not receiving appropriate care." The predatory nature by too many ill-advised and ignorant hospice owners to profit from the process of dying has forced good-hearted hospice professionals to take to social media to artificially reshape the image of hospice.

For the patients enrolled in hospice under the auspices of the huge corporate operators, there will be no improvement in care until there is an in-depth examination of the financial side of the industry. The discoveries in the report might help policymakers to develop stricter regulations in regard to the infusion of professional investment in the hospice space.

The OIG report also called for transparency on many levels: first, it would help consumers if the CMA made all of the family survey results and the complaint data public. And second, there should be laws in place to force for-profit companies to make public any changes in ownership. It is the only way the industry can detect those who are in the senior-care business for the wrong reasons. Finally, we must provide remediation for inexperienced providers and instill a ranking system to differentiate between the good, the average, and poor providers. We need a good, old-fashioned Angie's List of hospice providers in priority of excellence to poor.

As disheartening as it was to read this national report, sections of the report corroborated my experience with Hospice Advantage after it was purchased by the NYC Equity firm in 2012. And because of the change in our mission during that period, I witnessed many of our best clinicians leave only to be replaced by inexperienced and poorly-trained staff.

An AARP article on the current state of profiteering in hospice care written by author Christina Ianzito reiterated, "The OIG certainly doesn't want people to avoid hospice. Deputy Regional Director Inspector General Nancy Harrison said, 'It's an important benefit and can bring great comfort and ease the burden for recipients and their families during a difficult time. That's what it is created to do, and why there are real consequences when the services don't live up to their promises.'"

Next Steps

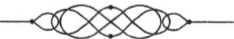

IN 2019, PROFESSIONALS WHO STUDIED AGING WERE CONCERNED that "too many for-profit hospices were gaming the system." That was a worry of Susan Enguidanos, an associate professor in the Leonard Davis School of Gerontology at USC. "It is true that healthcare has become corporatized to an almost unrecognizable degree in both the hospital sector and in hospice."

So where does that leave hospice care?

The end-of-life health specialty has been allowed to grow into a *commercial enterprise*, into an end-of-life *industry*, and into an ingenious *opportunity to acquire wealth* for profiteers. Hospice care has been allowed to be swallowed up by corporate and conglomerate businesses that trade on the New York Stock Exchange and Nasdaq. I cannot stress it enough: too many dying patients have become commodities, merely products in a business portfolio.

A hospice has only one chance to get the dying process right. A patient cannot have a 30-day trial period. Because dying patients depend on their hospice provider to always act in their best interest, a provider who is driven by a profit motive automatically possesses a conflict of interest.

However, Congress is starting to wake up and legislative reforms are being discussed and formulated. But not quickly enough. At the federal and state level, agencies need to monitor the growth of hospice companies and place moratoriums on licensing until inspectors can get a handle on what is occurring.

An article titled "Key Trends That Will Shape the Hospice Industry in 2023" was featured in *Hospice News* on December 13, 2022. Editor Jim Parker listed the changes that might help some of the current problems in the industry: "Government oversight of hospice providers will tighten this year; development of a new payment model; a redesigned survey process; the installation of a hospice complaint line from which the public can report issues to CMS; a newly installed Special Focus Program (SFP) with the designated power to enforce penalties; and a new OIG audit of hospices on their eligibility processes and violations of the False Claim Act."

Another obstacle to sweeping change in the senior care and hospice industry is persuading lawmakers and the public to make a priority of hospice care and quality nursing homes. The biggest underlying problem is that despite the billions of dollars that the United States spends on the system meant to care for the elderly, not enough is invested on the salaries of the caregivers. The unprecedented labor shortage in hospice, senior care, and in hospitals is the lack of fair compensation.

The rallying cry—if you pay them, they will apply—is a logical axiom.

The pandemic didn't necessarily contribute to the dysfunction of nursing homes and the hospice sector; it only revealed a flawed system. It started to deteriorate before I started working in skilled-nursing facilities in 2008. Low pay, tough working conditions, and long hours fueled a high-turnover rate which made it difficult to fill positions even before COVID-19 spread across our country.

A friend who works in the senior-care industry summarized it this way: "The chronic failure to value the work of hands-on caretaking in American nursing homes, and hospice at-home, and thereby compensate it, has helped to accelerate the loss of dignity for the elderly."

According to experts, the devastation wrought by COVID-19 and the public attention it has drawn to America's nursing home crisis and, therefore, hospice care (which is mostly delivered in nursing homes) have created an opportunity for far-reaching changes targeting the issues that left these facilities so vulnerable. Chiefly, funds from the government earmarked to bolster healthcare and end-of-life care for the elderly during that period did not trickle down to the patients, much-needed resources, and the certified nursing assistants. It went into the hands of owners and professional investors.

The typical American nursing home and hospice care are propped up by two programs: Medicaid, a public insurance system that is intended to support only the poorest Americans; and Medicare, a health insurance program for older Americans that offers nursing homes more lucrative short-term payments. This is the business model that the pandemic blew up.

Medicare is also the program that pays for most hospice services. The federal government sounded the alarm about the decline in good, consistent hospice care in its 2019 OIG report. News stories suddenly surfaced across the country with families revealing their poor experiences with hospice care. I still receive calls and emails from consumers asking for advice while using hospice services. Calls that often expose negligence and incompetence. Obviously, families don't call me when hospice care is excellent, but I encourage them to do so, as I take such joy from hearing those positive stories.

Congress, in response to the pandemic, designated $21 billion in COVID-relief funding for nursing homes. But there was limited oversight, just as there is in the for-profit hospice industry and no requirement that the money be specifically spent on staffing or resident care.

The overarching problem with public money is a lack of accountability, which only increases during a crisis, like a pandemic. Hospice has the same problem: Medicare tax dollars pay publicly-traded corporations and investor-owned hospice companies to care for the dying with miniscule oversight.

As the nursing home and hospice industry have consolidated in the last fifteen years with more acquisitions by large corporations and Wall Street investors, the ownership structures and finances have become increasingly complex and muddled. Therefore, many for-profit owners have created an arrangement known as "related party" transactions that allow owners to reduce liability and control costs. Critics say the practice allows owners of hospice companies and nursing homes to profit in ways that don't show up on balance sheets.

Kaiser Health found evidence in both elder care and hospice sectors that links the use of "related party" transactions to lower quality of care. For-profit companies with such arrangements employ fewer nurses and aides per patient on average and are more likely to be fined for serious health violations and have substantiated complaints of jeopardizing patients.

What I know about finances and marketing would fill a thimble, but I believe that federal lawmakers must force the for-profit hospice industry to open its books before offering more taxpayer money. I'm convinced we need more transparency around the allocation of professional investments in medical care, in general.

Seventy-one million baby boomers are heading into their golden years and many will need some type of long-term care and eventually hospice services. If we fail to address the root problems of the for-profit companies that currently take advantage of the sick and dying, our problems will only worsen.

In addition, I believe that there are changes in the industry that can be made in three areas that will improve the overall experience of direct patient care and shore up the current tarnished reputation of hospice care. First, transition programs are crucial in the palliative care-hospice space. This level of care is ideal for patients with a life-limiting illness and significant symptoms but are not within six months of dying.

It is specialized and certified palliative care for chronically ill patients who need moderate pain management, symptom control, and curative treatments for comfort like my patient, Helen. Palliative patients can have a life-expectancy of at least two years.

Second, we need larger nonprofit hospice residences with more beds for patients deemed to be within four to six weeks of dying. As it stands now, many inpatient hospices only have enough beds for the patients who need acute care in the final weeks and days of dying.

And finally, the families that undertake hospice care in the home need more support and education from hospice providers.

Epilogue
The Moral of the Story

O NCE UPON A TIME, THERE WAS A YOUNG MAN WHO LOVED beautiful fish. He wanted to create something special for them and watch them thrive under his care. His aquarium setup went flawlessly. He chose the perfect place, the decorations looked fantastic, and he stocked the tank with a bunch of gorgeous freshwater fish. Beaming with pride, he rested his head on the pillow that night and counted guppies until he drifted blissfully to sleep.

But in time, something seemed off. He was sure he'd stocked ten neon tetras, but now there were only eight. When the third week arrived, he found only five tetras. It slowly dawned on him that something was amiss. There was a murderer in their midst. One of the newly-introduced fish (a predator) was snacking on his other beautiful fish. The predator had a huge appetite.

He wondered, *How did this happen?* After the fact, he had learned that some fish are not meant to mingle and will harm the other fish. Some fish were too big and strong, more opportunistic, and too aggressive to add as tank mates. It should go without saying that you don't want to mix predatory fish to a tank with fish that are vulnerable and easily preyed upon.

As pet experts always mention, the most important thing is to research all of the fish *before* you allow them to enter your aquarium, so you can better understand their motives and behaviors. Then you can protect the more fragile fish. While that might not eliminate all surprises, it gives you the best chance of a successful outcome.

I found this delightful essay on a website by author Eric Dockett about helpful hints for the care of fish for small aquariums that I thought might be helpful for my youngest grandchild. As I read it, I couldn't help but make some comparisons to my work as a hospice chaplain working for professional investors.

Since my experience with Hospice Advantage, I've always wondered why a foreign marauder was allowed to enter the pastoral hospice environment? Why wasn't anyone watching the careless introduction of ambitious investors to an end-of-life medical space? Why were there no safeguards, guidelines, or controls introduced? Every fish lover and marine expert understands that you don't casually unleash a green-spotted puffer fish, a leopard bush fish, or the red devil into an at-home aquarium. They do not mix well. The tank will lose its pH balance and life-giving environment.

No one was minding the "store" while dangerous opportunists encroached and then seized the hospice sector for decades—the infiltration of private equity and other professional investment into the end-of-life medical space. What is considered a *success* for investors is not considered a *successful outcome* for dying patients.

So now, all professional hospice stakeholders and members of Congress must back up, reevaluate, and decontaminate the hospice space.

Questions for the Chaplain

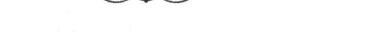

1. What is the work of an end-of-life doula and what is the difference between a doula and a hospice chaplain?

WHAT IS A DEATH DOULA? AT FIRST GLANCE, THE TERM might sound a bit macabre. Or perhaps you've heard the word doula used in relation to the birthing process. The term "doula" was developed in the 1960s to describe someone who is employed to provide guidance and support to a pregnant woman during labor.

This type of labor support has been utilized since ancient Greece. A death doula, also called an end-of-life (EOL) midwife, assists in the dying process. Both types of doulas coach human beings during major life transitions (during the start of life and at the very end). In addition, unlike hospice chaplains who are part of an interdisciplinary medical team paid for through Medicare, Medicaid, and some private health insurers, death doulas can be hired privately by families to companion patients in their homes and in nursing homes during the last months or weeks of life.

Doulas can be hired at any stage of illness to provide support and to help enhance a patient's quality of life before death. Therefore, the doula movement is a major contributor to the emerging field of palliative medicine. The well-trained doula provides emotional support, resources, comfort, knowledge, and insight. For example, they can empower a family and patient to reconnect during the profound experience of dying. They may also try to aid a patient in fulfilling their final wishes in an end-of-life (EOL) plan.

What is meant by an EOL plan?

Doulas facilitate the wishes of patients (if there is enough time) as I did in my practice. There is a lot for a dying person to ponder during this most profound period of transition and our culture tries to highlight significant milestones. Dying well is the primary, temporal landmark of our lives. It is a great achievement and blessing if it is anticipated and prepared for. It is a summons for family and friends to gather and bestow honor upon their loved one. It is a period to acknowledge and celebrate crossing the final threshold toward eternity; a time to remember, bury the hatchet, and grow spiritually and emotionally.

An end-of-life plan can help mark this occasion: it could include legacy planning, favorite music, room oil diffusers, memorable photos, art therapy, massage, reiki, pets, favorite personal items, religious rituals, prayer, beloved poems, family and friends, favorite food and beverages (if early enough in the process), basking in the sun and fresh air, a bird feeder stationed at the bedside window, a beloved hobby collection scattered about, and meditative environmental sounds.

Also, families and facility staff often need gentle guidance and education at the end of a loved one's life: for example, changes in condition, encouraging family members not to push eating as an antidote for their own grief or helplessness, and to understand that some loved ones describe seeing deceased family members at the end.

Most doulas come to the profession with backgrounds and experiences from a variety of careers which is valuable at the deathbed. They are not medical providers nor a part of the hospice disciplinary team, but are trained to minister in conjunction with them or independently. Some progressive hospice providers who understand the wisdom of partnering with the doula movement testify to the benefits for patients, families, and staff of that professional collaboration.

The doula movement has made great strategic and organizational strides in the last few years: it has trained more than 2,600 individuals and hospital staff in the last three years through the International End-of-life Doula Association (INELDA). The National Hospice and Palliative Care Organization has formed an End-of-Life Doula Council and hopes to involve its membership in volunteerism, as independent contractors hired by families, or as agency staff. Doulas, chaplains, social workers, and volunteers are trained to observe, listen intently, and create space for the immediate needs of patients and families in crisis. They provide a stable, objective, and calm presence during one of the most challenging transitions in life.

So what is the difference in training between a doula, a hospice volunteer, and a hospice chaplain? Hospice volunteers typically go through 20 to 30 hours of thorough training, but it is not as formal and extensive as the preparation for a doula. Some doula programs also provide training in light and energy work, an emerging practice for the dying and their families (I did some energy-balancing work with Katherine McCabe in Sturgeon Bay to understand its elements and merits).

There is so much potential in this discipline for those who are terminally ill or close to dying. Obviously, doulas and volunteers are crucial to a hospice team as vigil providers and a social/emotional presence for patients when the family cannot be present. They provide another "set of eyes" and extra help for the family.

For a hospice chaplain, the background required is extensive: a graduate degree in religious studies or a divinity degree from a seminary is the foundation to which layers of clinical practice in pastoral counseling are added. As well, many hospitals require the completion of four clinical pastoral education units to become fully-certified chaplains, which is equivalent to two years of post-graduate study (1,200 hours of clinical pastoral education, spiritual formation, and years of internships with the elderly and dying).

In addition, an ecclesiastical endorsement (from a religious institution) will take an additional six to nine months of paperwork and interviews. So, a chaplain brings to the dying bed expertise in the emotional, spiritual, and religious needs of a patient and their family. During my years in hospice, 90 percent of incoming hospice patients took services from a chaplain. All humans are spiritual beings, but not all human beings express their spirituality in a religious way.

A chaplain is trained to distribute Communion, plan funerals, deliver eulogies, arrange sacraments, explain scripture passages, offer spiritual direction and pastoral counseling, perform religious rituals, clarify and educate about religious issues, and discuss the theology of the afterlife. Chaplains must also be trained in grief work, forgiveness issues, and sacred music.

It's necessary to be familiar with the bibles of each of the three branches of Christianity (Orthodox, Roman Catholic, and Protestant) as families and patients are particular when it comes to the interpretation of the Sacred Scriptures of each denomination. Chaplains have also studied the five major religious traditions—Hinduism, Buddhism, Judaism, Christianity, and Islam—and their sacred writings.

So where does the doula profession fit in? The possibilities are endless. Suffice it to say, we need more professional doulas and volunteers to work in EOL care. Current data indicates that there is a "tsunami" of silver-and golden-agers nearing the end of life now and within the next two decades. Hospice professionals worry about the dearth of trained caregivers to accommodate the care needs of so many dying patients.

We live in a death-denying culture, but fortunately, there has been a positive death movement exploding across America in recent years and the doula profession is an aggregate of that fresh and healthy perspective. We are experiencing a groundswell, a change of thinking at a grassroots level that is calling us to view terminal illness and the dying process in a more natural, spiritual, creative, and holistic way.

Comfort around death is evolving with the development of platforms such as Dinner Over Death (DOD) conferences and Death

Cafés, which are popping up all over the map in urban areas. These pulpits facilitate conversations about dying or give those interested in being proactive about their own dying process a space to query, learn, ponder, and plan. The DOD program is partnering with the Cleveland Clinic and with Memorial Sloan Kettering Cancer Center in NYC.

The Death Café in Milwaukee is aptly coined "The Womb Room," which was started by Shantelle Riley to facilitate conversations surrounding death. Our western culture has separated death from the natural process of living and dying. The doula or soul midwife aims to return death to its sacred place in the celebration of life. When I speak to older adults about what they want at the end of life, they mostly articulate four requirements:

1. "I want control over how I die."
2. "I want a comfortable death."
3. "I want a death with dignity."
4. "I would prefer to die at home, but not be a burden to my family."

There are many exciting developments in the movement. Doulas are being prepared to offer multi-dimensional care to patients in hospice, their homes, senior communities, and large healthcare systems across the United States and Canada. Also, a Competency Badge (NEDA) can now be earned through a universal exam that assures patients, families, hospice providers, and hospitals of the legitimacy, excellence, and professionalism of doula training. It assures core proficiency, aptitude, and mastery.

The for-profit hospice sector complains that there are not enough chaplains, social workers, or CNAs to staff their agencies. However, the problem is that professionals are not being paid commensurate to their training and agencies overwork them. Consequently, this shift in priority and mission creates a huge space for doulas to be hired in homes and nursing homes. While hospice chaplains are mandated to minister within the strict requirements of Medicare and Medicaid, doulas are not constrained by corporate hospice practices and time constraints. The doula is an independent contractor, and that flexibility can only be beneficial to hospice patients and their families.

My readers often ask what the difference is between a social worker and a doula. There are seven different types of social workers. Hospice social workers help clients and patients navigate the planning for end-of-life care, connect to other resources and support, address crisis situations and stress, and educate families on how to advocate for themselves. They must have an undergraduate or a graduate degree in social work and be licensed.

I recently was privileged to interview two amazing women who are doulas. I met Deb Holtz on LinkedIn. She is a lawyer by trade and lives in the St. Paul area. She had performed a lot of advocacy work in government for people with disabilities during her legal career. She has a heart for healing. She's been a doula for four years and completed her training with Deanna Cochran's Quality of Life Care, LLC. She said that what she finds most satisfying about her work is watching patients make a peaceful transition.

Marggie Hatala, RN and certified doula trainer, received her training with Suzanne O'Brien and Doulagivers. She believes that Americans are not comfortable facing mortality. "What kind of a society pressures the elderly to live like millennials—running marathons at age eighty." She is the author of *Life as a Prayer*.

Where does one search for a doula training program? Four names and training centers kept surfacing for certified (EOL) Doula training:

1. Deanna Cochran, Hospice RN. Founder of Quality of Life Care Doula Training, LLC; founder of the EOL Practitioner's Collective; council chair for EOLDA; board member of the Doula Council for NHPCO; author, *Accompanying the Dying:*

Practical, Heart-Centered Wisdom for End-Of-Life Doulas and Health Care Advocates.
2. Tarron Estes, founder of the Conscious Dying Institute, Boulder, Colorado.
3. Suzanne O'Brien, RN, Doulagivers founder, speaker, and author in NYC. Board member member of the National Hospice and Palliative Care Organization (NHPCO). Founder of the International Doulagivers Institute. She assisted in developing the Doula program for some hospice providers.

It's important to know where consumers can find the services of an EOL practitioner. Information on training and how to find a doula directory can be found on the website of the International End-of-life Doula Association (INELDA).

Fees for doula services vary and it depends on the needs of the patient and family. Fees can be arranged hourly or contracted for an extended period. Doulas charge anywhere from $25 to $50 an hour. Many doulas utilize a sliding scale.

We can be better at dying comfortably in this country, so I would love to see legislation that takes the dying process out of the hands of corporate America. Dying should be tended to in the arms and hearts of nonprofit medical providers, for-profit providers who place patients as primary stakeholders, and within the emerging doula movement.

The EOL Doula Council within the NHPCO plans to evaluate the efficacy of doulas' collaboration with hospice services by conducting research to establish best practices for the future. The hospice industry desperately needs their assistance.

2. What are some of the nonprofit hospice providers in Wisconsin?

The Wisconsin Hospice and Palliative Care Collaboration is a partnership of the state's six leading nonprofit hospice and palliative care organizations: Adoray Home and Health, Agrace Hospice, Hospice Alliance, Rainbow Hospice Care, Sharon S. Richardson Community Hospice, and Unity Hospice.

In addition, AccentCare Hospice; Aurora Zilber Family Hospice & Hospice at Home; Cornerstone Hospice; Gundersen Health System Hospice; Horizon Home Care and Hospice was formed by Froedtert Community Hospitals, Columbia St. Mary's, and Lutheran Memorial Hospital; Luther Manor Retirement Community Hospice Care; ProHealth AngelsGrace Hospice; and St. Camillus Retirement Community Hospice Care.

It might be helpful to know that AccentCare Hospice Foundation is a nonprofit charitable institution that offers hospice patients financial assistance to meet needs not covered by traditional hospice benefits.

Acknowledgements

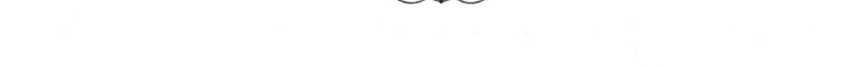

While my name is the only one on the cover, I am grateful to so many people for their assistance on this project. My book would not exist without them. Many folks who have inspired and mentored me throughout my life have set me on the path toward the writing of this hospice narrative.

My mother was the first role model on the joy of writing. So many people enjoyed her humorous and inventive letters typed monthly at the kitchen table.

I owe a debt of gratitude for the excellent education I received in writing, speaking, critical thinking, service, social justice, and leadership opportunities at the former St. Joseph Academy High School (now Notre Dame Academy) in Green Bay, Wisconsin; St. Norbert College in De Pere, Wisconsin; and Cardinal Stritch University in Milwaukee. The impact from the extraordinary teaching by nuns, priests, and lay educators alike was far-reaching and affected how I conducted my life.

From the beginning, as I sat in Laurie Scheer's workshop at UW-Madison, "On How to Draft a Book Proposal," she was a fervent believer in this topic and in my ability to write it. Her expertise and support in the last few years have been immeasurable on finishing what I started.

The craft of writing well is a process of study, practice, self-reflection, mindfulness, humility, and making sacrifices. Trying to find a publisher is an act of unending patience and courage. It also helps to read a lot of good books. The genesis of my chapters transpired at The Clearing Folk School in Door County with writing coach and author Judy Bridges, and at her Red Oak Writing studio in Milwaukee. And I am thankful to the dedicated writers whose paths I crossed at the Red Oak Writing Group under the guidance of author and creative writing instructor Kim Suhr. I am also grateful for the progress I made on my manuscript during a seven-day residency with Jerod Santek, executive director of Write On, Door County.

I owe an enormous debt to a group of talented editors, journalists, and authors who had a hand in polishing multiple drafts: Stacy Juba, Lauren Wiseman, Greg Peck, and Rev. Larry Patten. Kudos to Valerie Biel who is my website designer extraordinaire and supported me when I began this narrative in earnest five years ago.

And where would I be without the endorsement of Greg Schneider who wrote my foreword. He is a speaker, author, CEO, executive director, and founder of the Heal Project. Greg spends time as a volunteer caregiver and harpist for numerous hospices in California. He was selected by Johns Hopkins University to be a member of the Interdisciplinary Palliative Care Delegation to China and Tibet in 2006. Also, Greg founded the Hospice Volunteer Association (HVA), which is now the world's leading association for hospice volunteers and managers.

I owe a world of debt to my family, and former hospice and theology colleagues that offered to slog through early drafts and give constructive feedback. I love all of you for your helpful contributions: Laura Kukowski, CEO at Badger Hospice in Brookfield, Wisconsin; religion educator Karen Streich; Ingrid Klass Torinus, author of *Who Are You Times Two*; registered nurses from Hospice Advantage (HA) Millie D., Wani B., and Piper O.; Nathan Spielman, palliative caregiver with Optum Health; and sales representative at HA, Frank M.

So many friends and relatives encouraged me over the long haul: Kelly, Tim, Father Charles Hoffmann, Kathy M., Sue H., Terri C., Dona S., Patty, Jane L., Jean C., Paula, and Daniel McLaughlin.

Where would I be without the love, advice, and encouragement from my children who refused to let me quit when the going got tough. My artistic daughters Sarah and Annie contributed to my cover design; and my son Nathan handled my business affairs, read early drafts, and provided one final edit.

Leticia Hoisington: thank you for being an avid mental health advocate and for your tireless belief in my vision, talent, and inner strength. I owe you so much.

I also want to acknowledge the Wisconsin Writer's Association who published a version of my mother's hospice dying experience in their annual anthology, Creative Wisconsin in 2017.

And last, but not least, I am so grateful to the talented and creative team at Manhattan Book Group in NYC, who were a dream to work with and got me to the finish line in style; especially, Danielle, Madison and Lauren. Also, I want to thank MindStir Media Founder and CEO JJ Hebert for a publishing vision that provides opportunities for new authors with notable projects to get their books into the mainstream market.

Notes

Preface

Teno, Joan M. "Hospice Acquisitions by Profit-Driven Private Equity Firms." JAMA Network, September 30, 2021. https://jamanetwork.com/journals/jama-health-forum/fullarticle/2784807.

"U.S. Hospice Market Size, Share, & Trends Analysis Report By Location (Hospice Center, Home Hospice Care), By Type (RHC, CHC), By Diagnosis (Dementia, Cancer, Respiratory, Stroke), And Segment Forecasts, 2022-2030." Grand View Research, 2022. https://www.grandviewresearch.com/industry-analysis/us-hospice-market.

Angelou, Maya. *I Know Why The Caged Bird Sings*. Westminster: Random House, 1969.

On Call

Rumi. *The Essential Rumi*. Trans. By Coleman Barks, John Moyne. San Francisco: Harper One, 2004.

John

Churchill, Winston. https://www.forbes.com.quotes

Jung, Carl. "Fundamental Questions in Psychotherapy" in *Practice of Psychotherapy*, 239. Edited by Gerhard Adler and RFC Hull. Princeton University Press, 1966.

Rohr, Richard. *Falling Upward: A Spirituality for the Two Halves of Life*. Hoboken: Wiley Publishers, 2011.

Chestnut, Beatrice and Uranio Paes. *The Enneagram Guide to Waking Up: Find Your Path, Face Your Shadow, Discover Your True Self.* Newbury Port: Hampton Roads Publishing Company, 2021.

Blessing, William W. "Schizophrenia" in Handbook Of Clinical Neurology 156, 367-375. Edited by Andrej A. Romanovsky. Department of Human Physiology, Flinders University, November 17, 2018.

Collins, Suzanne. *The Hunger Games*. New York: Scholastic Publishing, 2008.

Christ in the Wilderness. 1872. Painted by Russian artist Ivan Kramskoi.

de la Cruz, Juan. "Dark Night of the Soul." c. 1579.

Spirituality and Religion

Wolfelt, Alan D. *The Handbook for Companioning the Mourner: Eleven Essential Principles*. Shippensburg: Companion Press, 2009.

Graham, Stephen. *The Gentle Art Of Tramping*. Bloomsburg Publishing: Oxford, January 2008.

Rohr, Richard. *The Universal Christ*. Convergent Books: Colorado Springs, Colorado, March 5, 2019.

A Day Away From Death

Potawatomi History. Milwaukee Public Museum. https://www.mpm.edu>I CW-152

Martha

Kushner, Harold. *When Bad Things Happen to Good People*. New York: Schocken Books, 1981.

What's In A Name

The Catholic Study Bible. Edited by Donald Senior, John Collins, and Mary Ann Getty. London: Oxford University, 2016.

Mowinckel, Sigmund. "The Name of Moses." *Hebrew Union College Annual* 32, 121-133. College Union College Press, 2016.

Matthew: 23:37. The Catholic Study Bible. Edited by Donald Senior, John Collins, Mary Ann Getty. London: Oxford University Press.

Bolz-Weber, Nadia. "A Mother Hen God." Center for Action and Contemplation. https://cac.org/daily-meditations/a-mother-hen-god-2022/03/28.

Nature of the Divine

Catherine of Siena Quotes. Https://www.azquotes.com

Visions and Signs

Williams, Margery. *The Velveteen Rabbit*. New York: George H. Doran Company, 1922.

The Gold Mine

Himmel, Sheila and Fran Smith. *Changing The Way We Die: Compassionate End-of-Life Care And The Hospice Movement.* Hoboken: Viva Editions, 2013. 149-166. Author permission granted to use material in chapter twelve.

Or, Amy. "Sentinel Capital Partners Takes Majority Stake in Hospice Advantage." Wall Street Journal. January 3, 2013. https://www.wsj.com.articles.

McNulty, John. "Sentinel Capital Partners Sells Hospice Advantage." Private Equity Professional. October 9, 2015. https://www.peprofessional.com>blog.

Leone, Gina. "Hospice Advantage Acquired by Compassus." Boston: Provident Healthcare Partners, 2004. https://www.providenthp.com/wp-content/uploads/2020/02/Hospice-Advantage-Compassus-Press-Release.pdf.

Edney, Anna. "Private Equity is Piling Into Health." Bloomberg.com. Bloomberg, September 27, 2022. https://www.bloomberg.com/news/newsletters/2022-09-27/private-equity-is-piling-into-health.

Knickerbocker, Kelly. "What Is Private Equity And How Does It Work? 12/22/2022 PitchBook Data. www.pitchbook.com.

No Place Like Home

Farmer, Blake. "Patients Want To Die At Home, But Home Hospice Can Be Tough On Families." National Public Radio. January 21, 2022. https://www.npr.org.

Kleiman, Arthur. "On Caregiving." Harvard Magazine, 2010. https://www.harvardmagazine.com/2010/07/on-caregiving.

How to Find a Trustworthy Provider

Medicare. gov. https://www.medicare.gov/care-compare/providerType-Hospice.

America's Health Rankings. "Senior Report 2019." United Health Foundation, 2019. https://assets.americashealthrankings.org/app/uploads/ahr-senior-report_2019_final.pdf.

Qualities of a Reputable Provider

Nitkin, Karen. "Drawing Conclusions." *Dome*. Baltimore: Johns Hopkins Medicine family, 2023.

Gray, Nathan. "Op-Comic: The Perils of a Profit Motive in Hospice Care." https://www.latimes.com/opinion/story/2023-02-05/hospice-agency-for-profit-nonprofit.

Cheney, Christopher. "Not-for-Profit Hospices Outperform For-Profit Hospices in Care Experiences, Study Finds." Health Leaders, February 27, 2023. https://www.healthleadersmedia.com/clinical-care/not-profit-hospices-out-perform-profit-hospices-care-experiences-study-finds.

Dying for Dollars

Himmel, Sheila and Fran Smith. *Changing The Way We Die: End of Life Care and The Hospice Movement*. Hoboken: Viva Editions, 2013. 149-151; 158-159; 161.

"Sentinel/Hospice Advantage/Healthcare/Private Equity." https://www.sentinelpartners.com.

Braun, Robert Taylor, David G. Stephenson, and Mark Aaron Unruh. "Acquisition of Hospice Companies by Private-Equity Firms and Publicly-Traded Corporations." National Library of Medicine, National Center for Biotechnology Information. Jama Internal Medicine 181, no. 8 (May 2021): 1113- 1114. https://www. ncbi.nlm.nih.gov/pmc/articles/PMC8094028/.

Parker, Jim. "PE Firm Acquires Comfort Hospice & Palliative Care." Hospice News, May 6, 2019. https://hospicenews.com/2019/05/06/private-equity-firm-acquires-comfort-hospice-palliative-care/.

Weak Oversight Breeds Neglect

Hawryluk, Markian. "Hospices Have Become Big Business for Private Equity Firms, Raising Concerns About End-of-Life Care." KFF Health News. August 1, 2022. https://kffhealthnews.org/news/article/hospices-private-equity-firms-end-of-life-care/.

The US Government Sounds the Alarm

"2019: Vulnerabilities in Hospice Care." HHS Office of Inspector General, last updated January 31, 2022. https://oig.hhs.gov/newsroom/media-materials-2019-hospice/.

Ianzito, Christina. "Many Hospices Offer Medicare Recipients Substandard Care." July 9, 2019. Article for AARP Magazine. www.feeds.aarp.org.

Chiedi, Joanna M. "Safeguards Must Be Strengthened To Protect Medicare Hospice." HHS Office of Inspector General, July 3, 2019. https://www.oig.hhs.gov/oei/reports/oei-02-17-0021.asp.

Stevenson, David, Emily Krone, and Robert Gambrel. "Tracking the Impact of Ownership Changes in Hospice Care Provided to Medicare Beneficiaries: Final Report." Office of the Assistant Secretary for Planning and Evaluation, Nov 30, 2018. https://aspe.hhs.gov/reports/tracking-impact-ownership-changes-hospice-care-provided-medicare-beneficiaries-final-report.

Poston, Ben and Kim Christensen. "'Large-scale Fraud' and lax oversight plague California's hospice industry, audit finds." *Los Angeles Times*, March 29, 2022. https://www.latimes.com/california/story/2022-03-29/fraud-lax-oversight-california-end-of-life-hospice-industry-audit-finds.

Center for Economic and Policy Research. "Preying on the Dying: Private Equity Gets Rich in Hospice Care." Eileen Applebaum, Rosemary Batt, and Emma Curchin. April, 25, 2023.

Next Steps

Parker, Jim. "Key Trends That Will Shape the Hospice Industry in 2023." December 13, 2022. https://www.hospicenews.com>shape-the-hospice-industry-in-2023.

Kirby, Hannah. "Milwaukee Area Death Cafes Provide Safe Space To Discuss Death, Grief." February 11, 2019. https://www.jsonline.com.

Hynes, Mary. "'Death Over Dinner' Brings Up The Most Important Conversation Nobody's Having." November 8, 2019. Las Vegas Review-Journal. https://www.reviewjournal.com.

Epilogue

https://www.pethelpful.com. Aug 12, 2022

Index

Accreditation Commission for Health Care . . . 223
a good death . . . 15,181
Allen of Bay . . . 147, 148, 149, 150
Andrews, Trey
    healthcare-focused private equity funds . . . 217
Angelou, Maya . . . 4, 190
Badger Hospice . . . 202, 203, 212, 250
Centers for Medicare and Medicaid Services
    basic payment and coverage structure . . . 128, 221, 222
Chaplain role . . . 36, 46, 98, 100, 120
Ciardi, Robert . . . 171
Clinical Pastoral Education (CPE) . . . xx, 15
Comfort Hospice . . . 218
comfort kit . . . 39, 45, 50, 53, 61
Community Health Accreditation Program (CHAP) . . . 223

Compassionate End-of-life Care And The Hospice Movement: *Changing The Way We Die* . . . xxi, 167, 173, 215
Compassus . . . 164, 171, 175
Dark Night of the Soul, The . . . 59, 71
Department of Health & Human Services (HHS) . . . 221, 231
    OIG Report . . . 223, 224, 227, 232, 235
Doula . . . 46, 210, 221, 241, 242, 243, 244, 245, 246, 247
    Definition of . . . 241, 246
    training and certification . . . 242, 243, 245, 246, 247
empathy . . . 71, 72, 163, 178
Enguidanos, Susan . . . 233
enneagram . . . 40, 41, 42, 140, 144, 186
Hell . . . 34, 43, 49, 137, 139
Himmel, Sheila . . . xiv, xxi, 168, 215, 216, 218

Hospice Advantage . . . 25, 26, 149, 165, 184, 186
hospice
    at home . . . 168, 181, 182, 211
    bereavement . . . 10, 225
    certification . . . xiv, 209, 222
    definition of . . . xiv, 10
    for-profit . . . ix, x, xi, xiii, 182, 197, 198, 203, 204, 205, 207, 208, 230, 233, 235, 236, 245
    interdisciplinary team . . . x, 5, 6, 12, 163, 170, 188, 197, 210, 241
    nonprofit . . . x, xiv, xv, xvi, xix, 178, 182, 196, 197, 198, 204, 209, 215, 228, 237, 247
    palliative care . . . xiv, 128, 172, 199, 221, 223, 236, 247
    vetting a for-profit provider . . . 197, 198, 204, 205, 208, 209
    volunteerism . . . ix, x, xi, xvi, 182, 210, 243, 250
Hospice Compare . . . 196
Hospice News . . . 217, 234
Institute of Medicine Report . . . 230
Joint Commission on the Accreditation of Healthcare . . . 223
Kaiser Health News . . . 224, 236
Kushner, Rabbi Harold . . . 110, 124
Lions Eye Bank of Wisconsin . . . 159

Los Angeles Times
    article on for-profit hospices . . . 231
Medical Record ADRs
    False Claims Act . . . 234
Mertz, Cory . . . 218
morphine . . . 17, 39, 45, 61, 65, 129, 130, 131, 141, 162, 163, 182, 183
    definition of . . . 39, 61
    cultural myths . . . 162, 163
Mountain Home Health Care and Hospice . . . 202
National Hospice and Palliative Care Organization . . . 224, 243, 247
Norwood Mezzanine Venture Capitalists (Wells Fargo Bank) . . . 172
pain management . . . xix, 53, 61, 101, 163, 164, 199, 210, 221
Parker, Jim . . . 217, 234
private equity . . . xii, xiv, xvi, 150, 170, 172, 174, 175, 183, 217, 218, 219, 230, 240
profit margin . . . xi, xv, 171, 204
Purgatory . . . 137, 140
Religious beliefs in my practice
    agnosticism . . . 46
    atheism . . . 46
    Christianity . . . 46, 244
    Indigenous spirituality . . . 82, 106

Islam . . . 46, 244
Judaism . . . 46, 244
Rohr, Father Richard . . . xx, 36, 37, 69, 101, 185
Rumi . . . 23, 24, 30, 35, 36, 52, 143
Saunders, Dame Cicely . . . xiv, 23, 65, 133
Sentinel Capital Partners . . . 164, 169, 170, 172, 175
Smith, Fran . . . xiv, xxi, 168, 215, 216, 218
spirituality . . . 45, 46, 82, 244
Stevenson, David . . . 224
suffering (the purpose of) . . . 9, 10, 54, 60, 90, 122, 124, 138, 140, 143, 163, 190
   emotional . . . 122, 123
   physical . . . 163, 190
   spiritual . . . 122
Thin Veil, The . . . 51, 66, 190
Towerbrook Capital Partners . . . 171
triple bottom line . . . 203
VITAS Hospice . . . 211, 212, 215, 216, 217
Wall Street
   hospice involvement in . . . 215, 216
Westbrook, Rev. Hugh . . . 222, 223

Printed in the USA
CPSIA information can be obtained
at www.ICGtesting.com
JSHW022238241023
50790JS00004BA/14